BASIC

ALSO BY COLONEL JACK JACOBS

*If Not Now, When? Duty and Sacrifice
in America's Time of Need*

ALSO BY DAVID FISHER

No One Would Listen: A True Financial Thriller
(with Harry Markopolos)
What Makes Business Rock (with Bill Roedy)
Up Till Now (with William Shatner)

BASIC

SURVIVING BOOT CAMP AND BASIC TRAINING

Colonel Jack Jacobs (Ret.)
and David Fisher

THOMAS DUNNE BOOKS
St. Martin's Griffin
New York

THOMAS DUNNE BOOKS.
An imprint of St. Martin's Press.

BASIC. Copyright © 2012 by Jack Jacobs and David Fisher. All rights reserved. Printed in the United States of America. For information, address St. Martin's Press, 175 Fifth Avenue, New York, N.Y. 10010.

www.thomasdunnebooks.com
www.stmartins.com

The Library of Congress has cataloged the hardcover edition as follows:

Jacobs, Jack, 1945–
    Basic : surviving boot camp and basic training / Colonel Jack Jacobs (Ret.) and David Fisher.
        p. cm.
    ISBN 978-0-312-62277-0 (hardcover)
    ISBN 978-1-4668-0244-5 (e-book)
  1. Basic training (Military education)—United States—Handbooks, manuals, etc.
2. United States—Armed Forces—Military life—Handbooks, manuals, etc.
I. Fisher, David, 1946–   II. Title.
    U408.3.J33 2012
    355.5'40973—dc23

                                                        2012009382

ISBN 978-1-250-03372-7 (trade paperback)

St. Martin's Griffin books may be purchased for educational, business, or promotional use. For information on bulk purchases, please contact Macmillan Corporate and Premium Sales Department at 1-800-221-7945 extension 5442 or write specialmarkets @macmillan.com.

First St. Martin's Griffin Edition: June 2013

10 9 8 7 6 5 4 3 2 1

To the men and women who have worn the cloth of the United States of America: thank you for your service, sacrifice, and comradeship.

—Col. Jack Jacobs and David Fisher

ACKNOWLEDGMENTS

The authors would like to acknowledge the cooperation of the many people who graciously granted us permission to use their material, including:

The documentary *Soldier Girls* (1981) by Nick Bloomfield and Joan Churchill. A DVD of this film can be purchased at these Web sites: Amazon.com, Play.com, Optimum, and MovieMail.

The documentary *Ears, Open. Eyeballs, Click.*, directed by Canaan Brumley, can be purchased at http://canaanbrumley.com/contact.html. Drill Instructor Staff Sergeant Mike Nichols, featured in this film, is a noted motivational speaker. He can be reached at SSgtNichols.com, where a variety of motivational materials are also available.

The documentary *Basic Training* by Fred Wiseman is available from Zipporah Films, One Richdale Avenue, Unit #44, Cambridge, Massachusetts 02140 or at info@zipporah.com.

Sergeant Michael Volkin is the author of several books, including *The Ultimate Basic Training Guidebook,* available at the online school Basic Training University. He can be reached at Ultimate-BasicTraining.com.

ACKNOWLEDGMENTS

Retired Air Force Master Sergeant Joe "Tuffy" Tofuri is the author of an acclaimed story of basic training, *Tuffy's Heroes*—Revised Edition, which can be purchased through the Army/Air Force Exchange Service, AAFES, at www.gipubs.com., and at Amazon.com.

A great variety of navy memorabilia, including cruise books covering the last eighty years and prints, can be obtained from Doug Kasunic, Great Naval Images LLC, 6815 Chadbourne Drive, Valley View, Ohio 44125. Visit GreatNavalImages.com for information.

We appreciate the cooperation of The Rutgers Oral History Archives, the Department of History, Rutgers University, for excerpts from an interview with Joe Salerno. This archive can be reached at http://oralhistory.rutgers.edu or by phone at 732-932-8190.

Some material was from the award winning solo show by performance artist and comedian Kahlil Ashanti. Kahlil can be reached at www.kahlilashanti.com.

Information concerning Daniel Landon's critically acclaimed play *Basic Training* can be found at CameronCompanyllc.com.

Jack Jacobs would also like to thank his lovely wife, Sue, for her inextinguishable energy, support, and understanding.

The authors would like to gratefully acknowledge the support of the entire staff at St. Martin's Press, Tom Dunne Books, especially Tom Dunne himself, our editor Peter Joseph, and the always smiling editorial assistant, Margaret Smith. We are both greatly appreciative of the efforts of Ivan Kronenfeld of New York's KKP who brought us together and Frank Weimann, President of the Literary Group, who helped turn our concept into reality.

David Fisher has fond memories of his own long-ago DI's at Ft. Leonard Wood, Sgts. Millard Deering and William Boyd, who reminded their troops to smile when the going got tough. He also knows that nothing good in his life happens without the continued support of his wife, Laura Stevens, their sons, Beau Charles and Taylor Jesse, and even the little dog who takes up too much space, Belle.

Going through Basic Training or Boot Camp is a unique individual experience that has been shared by many millions of men and women. Jack Jacobs and David Fisher would like to learn about your memories of this experience. Please share your favorite, or maybe not so favorites stories, with others who have done it, or with those would like to know about it. Please visit: www.Real -Basics.com, for an enjoyable, informative exploration of this initial phase of military training.

We landed in San Diego and they picked us up in a covered pick-up truck. The back was covered with a big piece of canvas so we couldn't see out. When we pulled onto the base in San Diego the truck finally stopped and they pulled back the canvas. All I saw were people hobbling around on crutches, people with their arms in casts, people wrapped in bandages. I couldn't believe it. Oh my God, I thought, what have I gotten myself into. Bootcamp is going to be a lot tougher than I expected it to be.

As I later discovered, for some reason the truck had stopped at the Physical Rehabilitation Platoon.

—**Richard Hubbard (Marines, San Diego, 1969)**

INTRODUCTION

Welcome to Basic Training

G ENERAL WILLIAM TECUMSEH SHERMAN might well have said, *"Life* is hell." We are all plagued by life's stresses. Late homework. College rejection. Overdue mortgage. Gray hair. Can't get rid of this creditor, this cough, the car's making a disturbing sound, etc. There is plenty of stress, and usually we don't have to look for it, especially as we get older, because it finds us. Even those who think they lead calm, simple, stress-free lives will eventually encounter a situation that is awful, overwhelming, painful, and does not go away by itself. It is guaranteed to linger and become more agonizing as time passes, in many cases to be overwhelmed by something else that seems even worse. If life is merely a method of replicating DNA, then the evolution of humans and their sentience seems like something of an opportunistic and sadistic prank.

Instead, General Sherman famously noted that of all life's challenges, it is war that is hell. Nothing in the world is as demanding or intense as armed combat. When faceless, unrelenting enemies are trying hard to kill you, all other problems fade into the invisible and insignificant distance. When it seems that every high-powered military weapon is aimed directly at you, and when the melon that used to be the head of your best buddy is disintegrated in a sickening pink spray just inches from you, the entire chemistry of your existence changes into something that can't be duplicated in any other laboratory of life.

In the surreal theater of armed combat, at the points of decision that face all warriors, there are only three things on which you can rely: courage, comrades, and skill.

Courage is rarely tested in civilian life, because there is nothing else like armed combat. It is not easy to predict who will be gallant in action, and so valor often comes from those who seem least likely to display it. War is a life-altering experience, and it forever alters the resolve of the least resolute and develops instant confidence in someone who had never demonstrated it before. In an instant, someone who had always harbored a fear that he would cower under fire is transformed by combat into a hero. The infrequent recognition of gallantry in action belies the fact that battlefield valor is a common occurrence, occasioned as much by the warrior's love of his comrades as by the threat facing them all.

There is some safety in numbers, and victory often goes to the side with overwhelming power, but at any specific point in war, success and survival are random and unpredictable, often hanging in the balance, with any outcome possible. Surely, survival is a triumph of chance over choice, for the randomness of selection on the battlefield is staggering. A spray of automatic weapons fire will miss one man and tear to pieces the warrior inches from him. In the midst of a firefight, whether you live or die is often the result of blind luck, the serendipity of fate, and the first derivative of this luck is fear.

Even in an automated world in which an enemy on the other side of the globe, blithely driving down a mountain road, can be blown to bits by a shirt-sleeved console operator nursing a cup of coffee, the majority of military service is full of opportunities to be scared. Actual armed combat, however, is a chance to be scared to death. "Courage is not the *absence* of fear," memorably remarked Bud Hawk, who received the Medal of Honor for his extraordinary heroism during the Second World War. "Having no fear would be the absence of intelligence. Instead, bravery is *overcoming* that fear," and it is the exigencies of the moment, the notion that action may prevail where inaction will mean certain death, that propel warriors to forsake personal safety and aid their buddies. This is something that can't be taught, but it is ingrained in a person's character when he arrives, and in basic training it is polished and prepared for use in the most demanding endeavors of his life. The extraordinary willingness and the skills of a human being to risk his life in the service of his comrades and the skills necessary to perform his military tasks to perfection begin at the beginning.

It is "boot camp" to the U.S. Navy and Marine Corps, but the U.S. Army's chronic lack of creativity in calling it "basic training" for once gets to the unromantic but essential nub of it. In every way—professionally, socially, psychologically—basic is the very beginning of an experience like no other. It is during this period of initial military training that a civilian—an otherwise ordinary person—is transformed into a warrior, that heroic figure whose exploits have saved fellow warriors, saved the day, saved the republic. Basic training is really a tiny period of time, just a few weeks, during which the lessons learned will shape a lifetime.

Of comrades it must be explained that nothing is more important. War is an alien environment, and the only real training for it is to experience it. Success in a war, a military campaign, or even a light skirmish is the result of concerted effort and, as with many other things in life, is not acquired with individual effort. Under conditions in which a single person's survival may well depend on the ability of a group to function as a cohesive organism, bonds are forged that can never be broken. The intellectual heritage of the archaic rules of military action is not Ralph Waldo Emerson but Benjamin Franklin, whose important guidance was delivered at the height of national stress, "We must indeed hang together, or most assuredly we shall all hang separately."

Finally, of skill it should be noted that basic training seeks to impart not the finely tuned professional capabilities of a journeyman but, instead, only some fundamental knowledge of the tools needed to learn more. The majority of skill as a warrior is acquired on the job: in the foxhole, on patrol, in the midst of terror and carnage. In basic, you learn that you should never travel down an unsecured road, but if you are foolish enough to travel down an unsecured road and subsequently survive the almost inevitable ambush, you will never travel down an unsecured road again. In basic, you learn the importance of keeping your rifle clean. The soldier whose dirty rifle jams while defending his position against a ferocious attack will, if he lives, forever have the most scrupulously clean rifle in the world. He will be fanatically fastidious about disassembling and cleaning his magazines and polishing every round of ammunition in them. In a very short time, combat turns callow, unskilled youths into mature, professional adults.

Courage, comrades, and skill, it is the foundation laid in basic training that inevitably will determine the strength of the entire structure. There is absolutely nothing comparable in American society to basic military training, nothing that offers the same challenges or rewards for a group of people only casually selected, and surely nothing that portends the importance of dedication to the task and the unpleasant consequences of failure. We proudly proclaim this country to be the home of the citizen-soldier, and what is extraordinary is that from the moment training begins, our citizens voluntarily surrender their liberty to become soldiers.

It is an irony of military life that those people on the front line and defending freedom must, of necessity, relinquish their own freedom. For those who have been dragged kicking and screaming into military service, as well as those young people who volunteered for it, at least some do cling to the comforting fiction that military life is like civilian life, except without room service. The large majority always understands that submission to authority is an implicit requirement of their service, and that includes authority over nearly every aspect of their person. They accept it as part of the price they pay for the honor of wearing the uniform.

But in one respect, initial military training may be the ultimate democracy: Every recruit, no matter the background, intelligence, or financial standing, is treated equally badly.

Recruits move suddenly from a flexible universe, in which they are permitted wide latitude of action on their own recognizance, into a confinement with a binomial character: There are tasks that must be accomplished, and there is only one way to accomplish them. You either hit the target, or you do not. You can either find your way from the deep woods to a specific, safe location, or, like Moses escaping from Egypt, wander for forty years and die before you reach your goal. You can either throw a hand grenade farther than the weapon's bursting radius, or you kill yourself and maim your comrades. For most tasks, there is little room for gradualism, partial credit, or failure, no provision for substandard performance that is accepted by the cadre with a smile, a pat on the back, and a friendly wish that you may do better when engaged with the enemy in actual armed combat.

Although no one knows the precise number, it is estimated that more than forty million men and women have gone through basic training and boot camp since World War I—and, as they proclaim proudly, survived it. Those millions of veterans and the additional

300,000 who negotiate basic and boot camp every year share an experience that lives forever in their memories.

My father had served in the Second World War, still fresh in the mind of the nation seventeen years after it ended, and I thought it was my obligation to serve as well. Rather than enlist after high school or submit to the vicissitudes of the draft, I joined ROTC in college, at least partially because it paid a derisively small stipend during the junior and senior years, and I needed the money desperately. My ROTC summer camp—except for the average educational level of the inmates, exactly like army basic training—was at Ft. Devens, Massachusetts, in 1965. Unlike trainees in basic or boot camp, which has often and with some accuracy been portrayed as a gallimaufry—rather than the traditional melting pot think of it as frying pan—of American archetypes: the intellectual, the hayseed, the criminal, the mental case, I went through training with people pretty much like I was: college students of some accomplishment and not a little irreverence. We viewed most of the instruction as essential knowledge but imparted in a ridiculously stilted, uncreative, inefficient, and pedestrian way. This made it less forbidding and instead more the grist for humor, and in many respects we thought we were in control of the system. We were the smart guys; we figured we were unique and we would invent ways of beating that system. And we continued believing that until we realized that we had become part of that system—and, in my case, I would remain a part of the system for much of my adult life.

Like the millions of trainees who had preceded me, and the millions who would follow me, the experience possessed the strong undercarriage of deadly seriousness dressed with the thin coachwork of comedy. The transition of becoming a soldier begins with the acceptance of the truth that at least some of what the recruit will do and learn during initial military training isn't going to make a whit of good sense, and a trainee who looks for logic in the day-to-day process is going to be terribly disappointed. For example, it is hard to discern the military benefit in scraping hardened wax from a linoleum floor with the dull blade of a mess kit knife, only to prepare the floor to be waxed again, and so we tend to deride such tactics as a misguided reversion to the dark time before humans became, as they are today, reformed and modern. In contrast with today, some of what took place decades ago in basic seems brutally stupid and troglodytic—and some of it was, particularly from the vantage point of a society that is today pure and enlightened. The training is a process designed to forge warriors from a society whose members perceive scant need for them and have not served themselves. Incredibly, at the end and despite the societal roadblocks, all the disparate, incongruous, and often foolish parts fit together.

Basic military training and boot camp are American institutions that have continued to evolve, and almost every aspect of the training programs has been examined and updated, but the experiences of trainees through the decades seem remarkably similar. For example, my father trained at Camp Crowder, Missouri, in 1943, and he never forgot the experience. Among those aspects that have endured are the live-fire exercises, which include the low-crawl and the grenade throw. As my father remembers it, "You had to crawl with your rifle for about one hundred yards while they fired .30 caliber machine guns with live bullets about three feet off the ground. The cadre would set off charges as you crawled, to simulate a real battlefield.

"When we went through it, one of the charges went off and sent bits of rock flying up into the air. A machine gun round hit one of the rocks and split it into pieces; one of those pieces hit a trainee in his leg and broke it."

This unintended consequence sounded pretty familiar to me. When I went through basic a generation later we spent one very long day learning how to throw a hand grenade. It isn't a particularly dangerous activity, especially if you have even limited experience throwing small, heavy, round objects. Except for the deadly explosions, hand grenades aren't much different from baseballs or rocks, and nearly every kid has thrown plenty of baseballs and rocks. We forty kids were supervised by two noncommissioned officers. The concept was simple: pull the pin, throw the grenade, duck. The only difficult thing is making sure you do it in that order. While one trainee was throwing, the rest of the platoon wasted time in bleachers quite a distance from the range. I was sitting there when one trainee threw his grenade, the fragments hit a rock, and the explosion propelled a small piece of shrapnel a huge, parabolic distance to the bleachers, where it struck and wounded the cadet sitting right next to me. One second, he was blabbing on and on about some nonsense, and the very next second, bits of teeth and a thick spurt of sunshine bright blood gushed from his open mouth and onto his chin. He looked like a predator that had been interrupted while feasting on a freshly killed elk. Shocked by the training's high level of realism and the improbability of being wounded without ever being in combat, he was led away to an ambulance, and although he was not badly injured, the dentistry bill alone must have been extraordinary.

Like most trainees before the advent of outsourcing food service to contractors, both my father and I served KP, and we never forgot it. "Among those things they had in abundance in the army were dirty pots and pans, boiling hot water, and an unlimited supply of manpower," my father says. "I washed a couple of the pans and couldn't get the things clean. I told the mess sergeant, and then *he* tried, and he couldn't get it clean either. So we got some GI soap, which was basically solidified lye, and ran hot water over the soap into the pan and put it on the stove until it was boiling, but we still couldn't get the pot clean.

"The sergeant looked at me and said, 'Ah, let's just throw it away.' Which is exactly what we did."

Like all additional duty, KP is supposed to be assigned from a duty roster, a simple chart that distributes onerous tasks equitably. However, it seemed as if I ended up on KP about a thousand times, and in any case much more frequently than anyone else. For some reason, I was always assigned to pots and pans and cleaning the grease trap, the two most hated, feared, filthy, and labor-intensive tasks in the mess hall. Favored troops got the plum jobs, of course, ones that did not require being hosed down and fumigated at the end of the day: stacking utensils or, best of all, mess hall orderly. Being an orderly consisted principally of standing around looking imperious, and all of those who were selected for this coveted duty shared many physical characteristics. Being tall, attractive, and having good posture were primary requirements. The small, hunched appearance of city kids eliminated many of us from consideration. Orderlies had to appear superb in a uniform. Some trainees look like they were constructed from birth specifically to wear a uniform, with the countenance of a snappy but guileless doorman. The rest of us looked like green laundry bags filled with door knobs or auto parts and were unsuitable for display.

As for the pots that were the objects of my labors: These were enormous vessels, and they looked big enough to boil whole animals or five hundred pounds of potatoes in them. Just like my father two decades earlier, my job was to clean them. As for him, they were impossible to clean. After several grueling wrestling matches with the pots, even armed with the good intention of doing my duty but failing totally in it, I realized that I needed some method to avoid the opprobrium that inevitably resulted from failing to get them spotlessly clean. I developed a strategy.

Unlike in real life and in military units in active service, where success is often the result of strategic and tactical flexibility, in basic training it is absolutely vital to develop a plan and, no matter what happens, stick to it. Stick to it like the congealed and burnt food stuck to the inside of a pot. Because the mess sergeant was never amused when he inspected pots that were not scrupulously clean, my objective was to insure that he never inspected them. After a moderately lousy job cleaning the largest pots, I'd set them on the floor and create a kitchenware *matryoshka,* nesting into them ever smaller pots, which were much easier to clean to the surgically antiseptic standard required. If the mess sergeant wanted to examine the big pots, he had to lift out many smaller ones, and I guessed correctly that he had little inclination to do so. I relied on the lassitude that affects most humans, an assumption, regrettably, that is valid in most endeavors.

I remember very clearly that, when I went through my initial military training, our platoon spent a great deal of time bellyaching about the idiocy of our leaders and the absurd tasks we were required to perform. It was difficult to discern the presence of an intelligent life form behind some of the vapid instructions we received, and no matter how hard we tried, the logic eluded us. If *we* were in command, we insisted, the situation would be quite different. We would treat troops properly, never waste precious time, and conduct training in a logical manner. Wouldn't we?

Then in 1968 I was assigned to Ft. Benning and put in command of an Officer Candidate Training company, and it was there I learned that nobody is immune to stupidity.

Many of the troops for whom I was responsible were seasoned

NCOs who had served in combat in Vietnam, E-6s and E-7s who would eventually go back to Vietnam as officers. The rest were college graduates who had enlisted specifically to go to OCS. All in all, this was a pretty competent group. There were three phases to this six-month course, and after completing the introductory and intermediate phases, trainees received blue helmets and blue ascots and became senior candidates.

In the middle of the night before they "turned blue," we cadre would wake them unceremoniously and order them out of their bunks with their foot lockers—their very heavy foot lockers. We'd make them stand in formation, at attention, in their underwear, foot lockers on their straining shoulders. It was all the more useful if the weather was cold and foul, and a driving rainstorm was always preferred. Then we would order them back into the barracks to change into their fatigue uniforms, leaving the footlockers behind. Now for the brilliant, mature, laudable part: While the candidates were upstairs, we'd peel the nametags from the footlockers and then stack the now unidentifiable boxes into a huge pile.

There was a good reason for doing this: We wanted to. Now, why we thought it was amusing remains beyond my comprehension. If there was a lesson to be learned, it was that these trainees, who by this time were feeling quite good about themselves because they were about to become seniors, were still trainees. Or perhaps that wherever you are in the military—or indeed any large bureaucratic organization—there will always be somebody in higher headquarters who will screw with you, just because he can.

Everyone who has been through initial military training will recognize with wry and perhaps fond understanding the stories in this volume. Paradoxically, they are simultaneously both unique and universal. Anyone about to go through training after reading this book will have some grasp of what he is about to endure. Those people who neither went through training nor will ever go through training will appreciate what they've missed.

This book is a celebration of basic military education, an experience shared by generations of Americans, a story told mostly through the articulated memories of men and women who have gone through it. There is a scene at the beginning of the great World War II movie *12 O'Clock High* in which the actor Dean Jagger walks down an abandoned airstrip overgrown with weeds, while in his mind he hears the roar of aircraft engines taking off. Then he looks through the broken window of the abandoned officers' club, and hears all the hoopla of that time of his life and is transported back into it. But more than his practical senses, his is the memory of emotion, a time when he was young, anything was possible, and the stakes were high. Basic training and boot camp are remembered the same way by most veterans, not for the tedium, the repetition, the ridiculous tasks, or the nonsensical rules and punishment, but rather for the people and the humor and the struggles they endured, and for their own ability to achieve more than they ever dreamt possible.

Welcome to basic training.

—Col. Jack Jacobs

If It Moves, Salute It: Welcome to Initial Military Training

You're in the army now, you're not behind a plow;
You'll never get rich, by digging a ditch
You're in the army now.
—traditional army marching chant

Congress judging it of the greatest importance to prescribe some invariable rules for the order and discipline of the troops, especially for the purpose of introducing an uniformity in their formation and maneuvers, and in the service of the camp: ORDERED, That the following regulations be observed by all the troops of the United States, and that all general and other officers cause the same to be executed with all possible exactness.

—In Congress, 29 March 1779, By Order, John Jay, President
(the beginning of basic military training)

"I am Gunnery Sergeant Hartman, your senior drill instructor. From now on you will only speak when being spoken to. The first and last words out of your sewers will be, sir! Do you maggots understand that?"

"Sir, yes Sir!"

"Bullshit. Sign off like you got a pair."

"Sir! Yes Sir!"

"If you ladies leave my island, if you survive recruit training, you will be a weapon. You will be a minister of death praying for war. But until that day you are pubes. You are the lowest forms of life on earth. You're not even human fucking beings. You're nothing but unorganized grab ass of amphibian shit. Because I am hard you will not like me but the more you hate me the more you will learn."

—from the movie *Full Metal Jacket*

THERE IS NOTHING AT all that compares to basic training. It's a period of several weeks during which civilians are transformed into soldiers, sailors, Marines, and airmen. There is no way to prepare for it. Those men and women who have been through basic will never forget it, and those people who haven't experienced it can't imagine it.

It's serious business, as Joseph Salerno learned on his first day at Camp Wheeler in 1943. "Right from the start they told us the theme was simple, 'You either learn to kill or you're going to be killed.'" Former Marine commandant David M. Shoup once accurately summed up the job of training depots, which, he said, were supposed to "receive, degrade, sanitise, immunise, clothe, equip, train, pain, scold, mould, sand, and polish."

As Brian Dennehy (Marines, Parris Island, 1969) explains, "Boot camp provides basic military training, but the real point is to indoctrinate you into a new way of looking at the world. The Marine Corps has a tradition of a very tough boot camp process. They are exposing you for the first time to the basic military philosophy—what otherwise might be presumed to be very risky activities. During this time officers and NCOs will tell you to do things to which your normal reaction would be, Hell no, I am not doing that.

"The basic objective of military training is to teach you how to operate as a unit, to become primarily concerned with unit cohesiveness and protection and to respond automatically to a situation that will achieve some goal. Boot camp is an assault on your individuality.

"The first few days at Parris Island is a deliberate assault on your citizen sensibility. You don't get to change your clothes, you don't get to stay clean, you don't get to shower. Any obvious signs of individuality are immediately stepped on. It's noisy, it's loud, and there is always someone in your face with some type of verbal assault. Everything you do is wrong and has to be punished, you're in a state of confusion and you're always tired. All of this forces you to respond as quickly as possible to these chaotic commands without thinking. This is a way of finding those people who are going to have trouble getting with the program. 'Getting with the program' is an important phrase, but once you get into this system of noise and confusion it all begins to make sense. And after three or four days of this the real training begins.

"I remember telling a lot of kids when we were in the barracks at night, 'Hundreds of thousands of guys have gone through this. There's no reason why you wouldn't make it.' Most of them did, too. The one thing everybody learns in boot camp is how much you can take. For most people, that usually turns out to be a lot more than they believed."

The history of basic military training is incomplete and erratic. Generally though, the introduction of organized military training is credited to Chinese general Sun Tze, the author of *The Art of War*, at about 500 B.C. According to legend, King Helu of Wu hired

Sun Tze to teach the approximately 180 women living in his palace close order drill and the proper use of the dagger-axe. Sun Tze appointed unit leaders, and when the troops failed to follow his orders those unit leaders were beheaded—thereby setting the standard for drill instructors that any recruit can easily identify with.

The concept of drilling soldiers, teaching them how to march and maneuver in formation, dates back to the Roman Empire, when Roman generals discovered that the infantry moved more efficiently when everyone was in step. The object of training was to teach soldiers how to maneuver in step. The Romans even defined the length of one step and marched to the beat of a drum.

Basic training began unofficially in the United States in Valley Forge, Pennsylvania in February 1778 when General George Washington brought in Prussian officer Baron Friedrich von Steuben to instill discipline in his unorganized, rag-tag Continental Army. Von Steuben trained a company of 120 men in basic military conduct and drilling. Because he spoke no English, he recruited an aide to curse at the troops for him. Troops were instructed to march at a seventy-six-step per minute cadence, rather than the current 120 steps. In battle at that time, troops maneuvered as a single unit, and the army best able to coordinate its moves gained a significant advantage.

When von Steuben's original model company was trained to his standards he dispersed them throughout the Continental Army to train other troops. He then wrote down his lessons in the "Regulations for the Order and Discipline of the Troops of the United States," which has become known as *The Soldier's Blue Book*. As he wrote in chapter five: Of the Instruction of Recruits, "The commanding officer of each company is charged with the instruction of his recruits; and as that is a service that requires not only experience, but a patience and temper not met with in every officer, he is to make choice of an officer, sergeant, and one or two corporals of his company who . . . are to attend particularly to that business.

"The recruits must be taken singly, and first taught to put on their accoutrements and carry themselves properly."

In the Beginning There Was the Heaven, the Earth, and the Drill Sergeant

EVERY MILITARY CAREER BEGINS when the recruit raises his or her right hand and takes the Oath of Enlistment. It is just about the only thing that every recruit throughout American history has in common. The moment a recruit's hand comes down he or she has surrendered almost all of their constitutional rights. They have entered into a new world, and the transition is sometimes difficult, often funny, but always memorable. The first such oath was created in 1775 for members of Washington's Continental Army. Enlistees had to affirm: "I _____ have, this day, voluntarily enlisted myself, as a soldier, in the American Continental army, for one year, unless sooner discharged: And I do bind myself to conform, in all instances, to such rules and regulations, as are, or shall be, established for the government of the said Army."

The current Oath of Enlistment became law in 1960. It reads: "I, _____, do solemnly swear (or affirm) that I will support and defend the Constitution of the United States against all enemies, foreign and domestic; that I will bear true faith and allegiance to the same; and that I will obey the orders of the President of the United States and the orders of the officers appointed over me, according to regulations and the Uniform Code of Military Justice. So help me God."

Few people know what to expect when they enter the military world. Olaf Casperson (air force, Lackland, December–January 1978–79) intended to use the military to get his education. "I had heard that the air force had veterinarians. Truthfully, it never occurred to me ask why the air force needed veterinarians, but I was hoping to go to school and become a veterinarian. At the processing center I was told politely, 'Son, we don't have veterinarians in the air force, but you don't want to do that anyway. That's a boring job. All those guys do is go around all day inspecting vegetables in the commissary.' So I asked about being a cook. But the recruiter looked at my aptitude test and put me into aircraft electronics. When I got home my Dad laughed at my story and said, 'They sure saw you coming.' It worked out very well, though. That became my career."

Susan Kincaid "Sparky" Allen (air force, Lackland, 1974) had a very similar experience. "I went in and told my recruiter I wanted to be a spy. Somehow he translated that to mean that I wanted to sign up for a six-year hitch in avionics."

There is a classic joke told about the first few days of basic training: In 1968 Richard Langsam, from the mountains of North Carolina, was drafted into the army. On the first day of basic training the army issued him a comb—and that afternoon the army barber cut off all his hair.

On the second day of basic training the army issued Langsam a toothbrush—and that afternoon the army dentist pulled out six of his teeth.

On the third day of basic training the army issued Langsam a jock strap—and the army has been looking for him ever since!

"I didn't have the slightest idea what boot camp was about," recalls John Langeler (navy, Great Lakes, 1966). "I was a college freshman twice, so obviously that didn't seem to be working out for me. I decided to join the navy to see the world. Before reporting I went to Brooks Brothers and bought two suits, several ties, and a leather suitcase. I wanted to be well dressed when I saw the world. When I got to the recruit training station there were fifteen other gentlemen there, each one of them holding a paper bag with a sandwich in it. I wondered, 'How are they going to get by without clothes?'

"It was pouring when we finally got out of the bus at Great Lakes. I was carrying my new suitcase with me. A senior petty officer came running, literally running, right up to me and pointed at it and said, 'Boy, what the fuck is that you're carrying?'

"It seemed obvious to me, 'It's a suitcase,' I said.

"His mouth dropped open. 'Boy, you call me Sir and what the fuck are you doing with a suitcase?'

"That seemed like a ridiculous question to me. What else is a suitcase for? I said slowly, 'It has clothing in it, Sir.' When he explained that the navy provides clothing for recruits, I pointed out, 'It's for the weekends.' I knew so little about boot camp I just assumed I'd need a jacket and tie for our weekend trips into Chicago.

"With that he opened it up and stared at it. Everything inside got soaking wet. The navy took it from me and shipped it to my home. My mother assumed the navy had given me a new suitcase so she just threw this one up in the attic—where all those wet clothes sat mildewing for several months."

The army even tried to change the MOS, military occupation specialty, of Audie Murphy, who eventually became the most decorated soldier of World War II. As he wrote in his autobiography, *To Hell and Back*, "During my first session of close-order drill, I, the late candidate for the Marines and the paratroops, passed out cold.

I quickly picked up the nickname of 'Baby.' My commanding officer tried to shove me into a cook and baker's school, where the going would be less rough.

"That was the supreme humiliation. To reach for the stars and end up stirring a pot of C-rations. I would not do it. I swore that I would take the guardhouse first. My stubborn attitude paid off. I was allowed to keep my combat classification; and the army was spared the disaster of having another fourth-class cook in its ranks."

No one knows how many millions of American men and women have gone through basic military training since the Baron first laid out his rules. In 2011 there were about eighteen million veterans in the United States. Although basic training, or boot camp as the navy and Marines call it, has been as brief as three weeks and as long as three months, depending on the needs of the military, traditionally it lasts between eight and ten weeks. After graduation recruits attend schools for advanced individual training in their military specialty.

Until 1918 each army division trained its own reinforcements, but the massive number of replacement troops needed to fight in World War I made that impossible and for the first time, central training depots were established. As the Center for Military History later reported, this was dismal failure. Many troops received less than a month of poorly conducted training before being shipped to the Allied Expeditionary Force in Europe and thrown completely unprepared into combat. They were sent to whatever units needed replacements and too often had not been trained on the equipment they were assigned. Their lack of preparation not only put their lives in jeopardy, it also endangered the troops they were assigned to support.

To make sure that mistake wouldn't be repeated, in 1940 "a system designed to provide a continuous stream of replacements trained in the necessary jobs" was established, although these replacement training centers weren't ready to receive recruits until March 1941. While basic and specialized school training was supposed to last thirteen weeks (it was eventually extended to seventeen weeks) after World War II began many troops shipped out after receiving only three or four weeks of basic combat training, often arriving in a war zone without ever having fired their primary weapon and sometimes even without being issued the necessary equipment. In the rush to feed troops into World War II combat zones, the established physical and psychological standards were very low. For example, when the army realized that too many recruits were being washed out of basic for "dental fitness," the dental requirements were lowered to the "ability to masticate the army ration." Meaning that if you could chew, you were in.

The centralized system wasn't really capable of training the number of troops needed for the war, so in many instances recruits were sent directly from a reception center to their assigned unit for basic training. For New Yorker Jerry Leitner (army, Fort Sill, Oklahoma, 1944) that was an artillery unit. "I was a Jewish college student from Queens. Sometimes they tried to match your interest with your assignment, but this was not one of those times. After I got to Ft. Sill they sent me to a large room, and hanging on the walls were photographs of the various types of field artillery, starting with the 75 mm left over from World War I right up to the 155 mm cannons. A lieutenant asked me, 'Anything here interest you?' I didn't know anything so I pointed to the biggest cannon, the 155 mm. He smiled, then said, 'Look, you're six feet tall and in good health, how'd you like to be in the roughest toughest group in field artillery?'

"I'd been in the army a week. I knew very little about anything, but I knew he was going to send me wherever he wanted to send me. So I said, 'Sounds good.' He gave me a slip of paper with a number on it and I got into a truck with a lot of other young people who knew as little as I did. Every time the truck stopped a sergeant would shout out a number and somebody would get off. That happened until I was the last one left. It was just after sunset when we got to my assignment. Mule pack artillery. I didn't have the slightest idea what that meant. It turned out it meant exactly what it sounds like; in terrain too rough for a vehicle, the mule pack artillery would break down a 75 mm cannon into pieces, put a piece on the back of a mule and if the mule is willing, get in front of it and pull it in the direction you want it to go. Maybe they thought with my three years of college I could argue with the mule.

"I learned a lot of things they didn't teach in college. For example, I learned how hard it was to scrape mule shit from that crevasse between the shoe top and the sole. I remember the warning we were given, 'You don't touch a mule in a certain place—or it will kick you into space.' And I learned how to properly load a mule.

"The unit was all southern farm boys and me. One night they put us in a truck and dropped us in the middle of the woods. 'Okay,' the sergeant looked at me and demanded, 'which way is north?'

"Are you kidding me? I thought. North? I was from Queens, New York, and I was standing in the middle of an Oklahoma forest in the pitch dark talking nicely to mules. And this guy wanted to know which way was north? I didn't have the slightest idea. I told him, 'Why don't you ask me which way is uptown.'

"After four or five days a lieutenant showed up and asked me seriously, 'Leitner, you got three years of college under your belt, what the hell are you doing with the mule?'

"I had been born and grown up on the streets of New York, so I had a lot of possible answers for that question. None of them would have helped my career. Instead, I just shook my head. 'Trying not to get kicked,' I admitted. He told me I'd been sent to the wrong place. That was the end of my career in mule pack artillery."

The new replacement training system couldn't turn out troops quickly enough to meet the battlefield needs, and by late 1944 had broken down. Once again inadequately trained and equipped troops were sent into combat, putting themselves and their fellow troops into danger.

At the end of the war it had become obvious that a better system of training was required. In 1946 the foundations for the current system were created. While the army has trained recruits at numerous different bases throughout its history, currently there are five training bases, with Fort Jackson, South Carolina, being the largest. All female recruits are trained at Ft. Leonard Wood, Missouri—known somewhat affectionately as Ft. Lost-in-the-Woods—and all army recruits, including Army Reserves and National Guard, go through exactly the same training.

Where to Begin

> You gotta get up, you gotta get up, you gotta get up this morning.
> —generally accepted lyrics to Reveille

F OR ALMOST ALL RECRUITS basic training begins at a reception station, where the formalities of processing recruits into military life are taken care of. While this period is commonly known as "zero week," it can take only a few days or last longer than a week, until enough new recruits arrive to fill a training company. Those first few moments, when the world changes, are always among the most memorable. "We got there on a bus in the middle of the night," remembers Mitchell Friedman (army, Ft. Leonard Wood, 1969). "Every person there must have been warned by somebody, 'Don't be in the front, but don't be at the back either. So when we got off the bus 250 guys began scrambling to be right in the middle. It was like the biggest game of musical chairs ever played."

That first day was just as chaotic when Michael Volkin arrived at Ft. Leonard Wood in 2001. "The first task on the first day was to get off the cattle truck with our three duffel bags of new gear and get lined up in alphabetical order. It would have helped if we knew each other's names. We didn't. We had no leaders so more than 200 recruits just stumbled around trying to organize ourselves in alphabetical order."

Once recruits manage to assemble in some form of order an instructor makes a welcoming speech, which Saul Wolfe (army, Ft. Dix, 1958) summed up as simply, "Your heart may be home with your momma, but your ass is mine."

Arriving at navy boot camp isn't any different. Will Cortez (navy, Great Lakes, 2010) explains, "It started calmly. We arrived at the airport and they put us on a bus. While we were driving to Great Lakes they showed us a video. Everybody was so nice, so friendly, telling us boot camp is a quick eight weeks. When the bus got to the processing center an officer asked, 'Are you guys ready?' We were all thinking, this isn't going to be so bad, when that same officer suddenly exploded. He started screaming, 'THEN GET OFF MY BUS! GET OUT! GET OUT!' We stayed awake for the next two days with someone in your face every minute. We walked around in a daze getting yelled at."

The history of navy boot camp can be traced back to 1881, with the founding of a training station on Coaster's Harbor Island, in Newport, Rhode Island. Prior to that, when sailors enlisted they were sent directly to their assigned ship where they would be trained while under way. There are various stories concerning the derivation of the term "boot camp"; while it is commonly accepted it refers to the white leggings, or "boots," worn by sailors during the Spanish-American War, a more colorful explanation dates to the early 1890s when sailors, who traditionally would swab decks barefoot, began wearing waterproof rubber boots, becoming known as "rubber boot sailors," or "boots."

Since 1993, when training stations in San Diego and Orlando were closed, the navy has trained its recruits at the Great Lakes

Naval Training Station, located north of Chicago, Illinois. Great Lakes was opened in 1911 when the first "boot," a man named Joseph Gregg, reported, and the station has become known by several nicknames, including "The Quarterdeck of the Navy," and more ominously "The Great Mistake." Ironically, although Great Lakes trains sailors for sea duty, it is located on Lake Michigan, thousands of miles from any ocean. In fact, it originally was sited there because it was close to the nation's railroad hub in Chicago, which made transportation to and from anywhere in the country possible.

The Naval Training Center at Orlando was commissioned in 1968 and graduated its final class in 1998. As Eric Dell (navy, Orlando, 1994) remembers it, "When I got to Orlando and stepped off the bus I think the drill instructors were particularly annoyed with my purple hair. It's fair to say I attracted some attention. Maybe a lot of attention. The first few days the drill instructors weren't allowed to physically exert us without our full medical test being done, so they resorted to other means of 'challenging us,' as they referred to it. My favorite was the night they made us hold out our boot-camp issued pens at arm's length and hold them there. These were just little pens. Never in my life would I have thought a pen could weigh as much as a small car. After several minutes of holding out that pen my arms were shaking uncontrollably and the weaker men in my group had started crying; I mean crying real tears.

"I shared a room at Orlando with eighty strangers. We were given two tiny desk drawers for our personal effects; stamps are considered personal effects for example. This room became the cleanest thing I have ever known. There was not one iota of dust present because that would cause us to do 'Eight count body-builders until you drop, and I am not kidding, one of you will drop.'

"I never thought for one second that I could possibly care so much about how I made my bed, whether or not it had 45 degree hospital corners, not a single crease and was pulled so tight that a quarter would bounce off it. They took inspections seriously there. One time our drill instructor thought we were treating the inspection as a joke so he invited drill instructors from other companies to come over to our barracks to help us redefine our love for inspections. They cycled us, that's an expression meaning exercise the crap out of us, for about three hours. Again I saw grown men crying, which became a theme."

The Naval Training Center in San Diego was commissioned in 1923, partially because the persistent fog covering the training facility then in use at Goat Bay near San Francisco made sailing difficult, which obviously would be a problem for the navy, as well as its proximity to the Pacific Fleet. San Diego eventually became the navy's largest training center. When it opened recruits spent their first three weeks there living in tents in the Detention Camp, which actually meant they were quarantined to prevent the spread of disease, but that name was changed after concerned parents wondered why their sons were being "detained" by the navy. It was reported in the camp newspaper that the one hundred–man training companies "competed against each other in sea bag and personnel inspections, as well as barracks cleanliness." Among the most popular training exercises was whaleboat racing, a team sport that taught seamanship—and rowing. A lot of rowing.

The Marines also have a training center at San Diego, in addition to the legendary Marine Corps Recruit Depot at Parris Island, South Carolina. Recruits trained in San Diego are often referred to as "Hollywood Marines," because of its proximity to the movie industry, while men and women who go through boot camp on Parris Island are sometimes called "Swamp Dogs," a reference to the less glamorous swamps and bogs that cover the sand flea–infested island. All female Marine recruits are trained at Parris Island. As Joe Lisi (Marines, Parris Island, 1969) explains, "You have to earn the right to be called a Marine. There is no guarantee you will make it through training and you are not a Marine until the end of boot camp. The Marine Corps is very precise about not calling a person a Marine until they have finished training, until then you are 'recruit' or 'private.'

"It is arranged purposefully that recruits arrive at night. When we got there a drill instructor came on the bus and immediately started yelling at everybody. We hadn't had time to do anything except sit there and already we were doing it wrong. The first thing he screamed at us was 'Get off my bus and get on my footprints.' Every single Marine recruit begins their career standing on those yellow footprints in the reception area. They are arranged precisely at a 45 degree angle, which is the proper way to stand at attention. No Marine will ever forget standing on those yellow footprints. After that your life is never the same again.

"One thing I remember is that the drill instructor suggested that it would better for our future health if we moved as quickly as possible getting off the bus—but he didn't say it so nicely. In fact, when he ordered us to get off that bus it became a mad scramble. People were pushing and shoving—and one of the people hustling to get off the bus fell and broke his leg. That was my introduction to Parris Island. I remember thinking, wow, if some guy broke his leg just getting off the bus, Parris Island is going to be a little tougher than I thought."

The first formal Marine training facility was established in Washington, D.C., more than two hundred years ago. In 1808 Marine recruits were trained in the "principles of military movement," which meant learning how to march in formation.

Marines have been training on Parris Island since 1915, six years before San Diego was commissioned. Marine Corps basic training is the most physically demanding of the services. The object is to create the toughest possible combat soldiers. Thomas Kilbride (Marines, Parris Island, 1980) explains, "In the Marines it's called boot camp, not basic, because basically it's a boot in the ass. I guarantee that during boot camp the instructors will find out each recruit's biggest fear, I don't care if it's water or heights, whatever it is, and make them face it."

The United States Air Force officially came into being in 1947 when President Truman signed the National Security Act, which combined the Army Air Force and Army Air Corps into a single independent organization. In 1942 the army opened the San Antonio Aviation Cadet Center in Lackland, Texas, and since 1946 all air force recruits have been trained at the renamed Lackland Air Force Base. From the very beginning, because the demands of the air force are different than those of ground combat troops, basic training has been less physically demanding in the air force than in the Marines or the army. "Air force basic training is nowhere near as strenuous or mind-bending as Marine or army infantry basic training," explains Paul Setmaer (air force, Lackland, 1977). "Basically, the air force wants to teach recruits to take direction and follow orders. There are physical fitness aspects, but in reality they want to see if you can pay attention and follow instructions because eventually a lot of recruits are going to be taking care of multimillion dollar aircraft and equipment. The first thing they do is try to weed out people who can't follow simple orders."

Paul Ehrman (air force, Lackland, 1965) remembers being assigned to the original barracks at Lackland. "If you were on the second floor you could see right through the floorboards to the first floor. At that time Lady Bird Johnson had embarked on a beautification of America program. People used to say that if Lady Bird Johnson really intended to beautify America the first thing she had to do was come to Lackland and burn down the barracks."

Diversity Will Never Be the Same: The Military Breaks Down Barriers

SERGEANT: Dig, soldiers, dig, dig down to China.

RECRUIT ROSS: China? I thought this war was in Europe. I've been working in the subway all my life. I never thought about the guys that dug it. But since I'm in the army I sure take my hat off to them.

RECRUIT YORK: Subway? What's this here subway you're talking about?

ROSS: You mean to say you don't know what a subway is? . . . Where you from?

YORK: Tennessee.

ROSS: Ain't you ever even seen a subway?

YORK: Ain't never even heared a one.

ROSS: You never heared? What kind of talk is that? Do they all talk that kind of English where you come from?

YORK: Well, there ain't any English people down our way. Just Americans.

ROSS: Look, a subway is a big hole in the ground, see. It goes for miles.

YORK: Straight down?

—from the movie *Sergeant York*

Often the trip from a recruit's hometown to basic is the beginning of a journey to another world. While much less so now than in the past, basic training has always brought together recruits from different parts of the country and exposed them to people, cultures, and religions that in many instances they had never experienced before. Tom Jones (army, Ft. Gordon, Georgia, 1962) "took a train from Pittsburgh heading south and they let us off in a tiny little hamlet in South Carolina. It was about 10:00 at night and there was a little bar at the end of the station. We realized there wouldn't be another train for an hour so I suggested we go get a beer. Everyone was behind me and as I walked in the door I saw a sign that read, 'Yankees, N——s, and GIs keep out.' I tried to make a joke out of it, saying to the guys I was with, 'Oh, shit, two out of three.' Then I heard the guy right behind me respond glumly, 'Three out of three!'"

Michael Volkin remembered being thrown together with "a bunch of people I probably wouldn't have met in civilian life. I was a typical white suburban kid and a lot of the people I went through basic with were there in answer to the simple question, 'Would you rather be in the army or in jail?'"

New Yorker Herb Cohn (army, Ft. Dix, 1963) was in a platoon with about equal numbers of northerners and southerners, and he explains, "On beer nights we used to buy bottles of beer for the southern kids just so we could watch them opening the bottles with their teeth. It never ceased to amaze us how they could do it, or how far a canine tooth could fly out of a mouth."

In the military, it is illegal to discriminate against anyone for any reason. It wasn't always that way. The services were segregated until President Harry Truman ordered otherwise, and there have always been clashes between trainees of different backgrounds. As one Drill Sergeant was reported to have explained to his troops on the first day of a new training cycle at Ft. Jackson, "I respect all religions. If on Sunday we don't have a church for you to worship here, then I will make a place for you to worship. If you are Wiccan I will let you practice your witchcraft in this back room you see behind me, just as long as you don't try to turn me or your battle buddy into frogs or put some other weird curse on us. I myself am a very religious person. For example I worship my M-16. Every Sunday I go to the church of M-16ism and worship the most badass weapon on the battlefield."

For some recruits basic training was the first time they met people who practiced different religions. As Richard Goldman (army, Ft. Jackson, 1968) explains, "I was a Jewish reservist from Long Island and several of the recruits in my unit were from the hills of Kentucky. One person I remember in particular had the bunk directly beneath mine. He was from a place called Sugar Tree Hollow. About the fourth night there I woke up and felt this hand on my head. I jumped out of bed and it's this kid and he's touching my head. 'What are you doing?' I snapped at him.

"He said, 'You're the first Jew I've ever met. We heard Jews had horns.' He was feeling my head to see if I really had horns. He wasn't being malicious, he was just curious. As happens when you go through basic with a guy, eventually we became friends. At the end of training I was going back to New York, but he was regular army so he was going to Vietnam.

"About a week before we graduated we were in the communal shower. It had a pole down the center of the room with shower heads coming out of it. There was a low wall down the middle and we stood on either side of that wall. This kid walked in and I saw that he had about six chains around his neck with every kind of lucky charm you could imagine. I was wearing a mezuzah, a long, thin silver charm holding a small piece of the Torah, around my neck. He pointed at it and asked what it was, and I don't know where this answer came from, but I told him, 'It's a Jew whistle. See, Jews have very acute hearing, we can hear things other people can't hear. When a Jew is in trouble he blows his Jew whistle and all the other Jews around have to come to help.' When he told me he didn't believe me I said, 'Okay, it's only supposed to be for an emergency, but I'm going to blow it one time, just one time.' I knew that my friends on the other side of the shower were listening to every word, so I put the mezuzah in my mouth as if it was a whistle and blew. Two of my friends came right around the low wall, stark naked, asking what the problem was. This kid was blown away, he thought this was the greatest thing in the world. So I took off the mezuzah and put it around his neck for good luck. A week later we were discharged and I returned to New York.

"That probably was a mistake. I knew he went to Vietnam. Several months later the Tet Offensive took place and I had this horrible thought of him crouched in a foxhole blowing his Jew whistle waiting for help. I never found out what really happened."

"We had people with us who had never worn shoes, literally," remembered David Jacobs (army, Camp Crowder, Missouri, 1943). "So they certainly knew nothing about Judaism. That became obvious when just before Purim the cadre put a note on the bulletin board announcing there would be Friday night Purim services. A 2nd lieutenant brought all the Jewish personnel into a room and told us confidently, 'I know it's your holiday, but it's also GI night when the barracks get cleaned. Believe me, it's okay not to go to services. Jehovah will forgive you.'"

When David Fisher was at Ft. Leonard Wood in 1969 one day at the beginning of the cycle the Drill Sergeants gathered all the trainees and separated them by religion. "There wasn't anything wrong with it. They just needed to know who was going to church on Sunday and who was going to 'Jewish church on Saturday.' They divided us into three groups, Protestants, Catholics, and Jews. Everybody joined a group except for one African American kid, who was standing there in the middle of the road all by himself. One of the Drill Sergeants asked, 'Son, what is you?'

"He replied, 'Musss-lim,' drawing out the word. This was 1969 when the only Muslims anybody knew anything about were the Black Muslims, a pretty radical group. A lot of people were frightened of them. So this was potentially a real problem for the Drill Sergeants. They obviously didn't know how to handle this. They huddled up and discussed it for a while, until finally one of them turned his head and asked this kid, as if it made any difference, 'Son, did you say Muslim, or Moslem?'

"The kid hesitated for a few seconds, then frowned and waved his hand, 'Oh shit,' he decided, 'I'll be a Catholic.' Then he walked over and joined that group."

When Val Nicholas was asked his religion, he remembers, "I'm Catholic, but I decided to be smart and I said I was an evangelical agnostic. The sergeant paused for a few seconds, thinking about that. Then he asked, 'Were you baptized in America?'

"'I was,' I told him.

"He nodded with satisfaction. That solved his problem. 'Okay then, you're an American Baptist.' So I had to go to the Baptist services."

Even before he gave up his mezuzah, Richard Goldman admits he used his religion to avoid duty and Saturday inspections. "I found religion in basic training. Maybe it's more accurate to say I invented religion in basic. At Ft. Jackson they didn't know anything about Judaism except that whatever we did we did it on Saturdays instead of Sundays. And that there were a lot of holidays with very strange names. It turned out there were especially a lot of Jewish holidays, because we made them up. 'Oh, Sergeant, it's a big holiday, Tish Shibon, and it's a day of rest. We can't do anything.' We came up with the most ridiculous holidays, but fortunately they always coincided with the toughest work days."

Ira Berkow (army, Ft. Leonard Wood, 1958) agrees that "It was amazing how religious basic training makes you. The Jews in my platoon became very religious people. Literally we were praying to get out of duty. Our Drill Sergeant figured that out and was pretty unhappy about it. So what he would do after we got back from synagogue was have us pick up rocks from one side of the road and bring them across to the other side. And then on Sunday, when the other guys were at church, we would pick up the same rocks and return them to the original side."

It wasn't only Jewish personnel who attended services, of course. "Everybody went to chapel every Sunday," remembers Anthony Bayse (army, Ft. Dix, 1989). "If you didn't go to church you were back in the barracks cleaning, shining your boots, mopping the floors, you were doing something. So everybody went to chapel.

"Besides, it was the only place where you could get some sleep. It was the one time during the week we didn't have the Drill Sergeants breathing down our necks. The pastor never objected. All anybody wanted was just a few minutes where we could sit down and not be harassed—and our prayers were answered in church."

Years ago, anti-Semitism and racism were rampant in the military, a place where the views across America were distilled and concentrated. "There was a problem with being Jewish in Texas during World War II," remembers Milton Pike (army, Camp Shannon, 1944). "When we did hand-to-hand combat practice, for example, I was usually the guy they picked to be the German." At Ft. Knox in 1945 Ralph Strauss had a similar experience. "I'd go out of the barracks and I'd come back in and my shoes were nailed to the floor. I found a box of corn flakes in my bed. They were a bunch of bastards."

At Great Lakes in 1966, "The southern guys just hated blacks," Tom Fitzsimmons says flatly. As a New Yorker he had never before been exposed to rabid racism. "It was amazing. Some of the people from the Deep South were vicious. If they were smoking a cigarette when they walked by a black man, for example, they would stick it in his arm. I got cornered one day by a group of guys from Tennessee who warned me that if I didn't stay away from the black trainees, and believe me that was not the way they referred to them, I would suffer the same consequences they did. That was it, for me. I drew a line in the sand.

"But they had the system going for them. We had one Drill Instructor from the Deep South who basically hated the New York City guys. We had an inspection the afternoon after I had been warned, and this DI knew right where to go. He looked me in the eye, reached into my pocket, and found some coins that had obviously been planted there by the southerners. He wrote me up, and I was ordered to walk guard duty on the Dumpsters for hours, every freezing cold night. They made life as hard as possible for all of us."

Of course, Adam Mandlebaum (air force, Lackland, 1970) managed to find the humor in a sensitive situation. "We had a few black trainees with us, and once they got to know the New Yorkers they knew when we were kidding. They called me 'The Rabbi' because I was the only Jewish guy in our outfit. My bunk was next to one of these black guys. So one night I was shining my boots with a cotton ball, and I held it up for him to see and asked, 'Bring back any memories?' Everybody laughed. Fortunately."

New Yorker Ira Fogel (army, Ft. Gordon, 1966) wasn't ready for the reception he received. "We stood in line for the first meal and they asked me where I was from. 'New York,' I said, assuming everybody was friendly. As I went through the chow line the first thing they put on my tray was shrimp. Then, right on top of the shrimp they put the potato. On top of the potato they put the vegetable, on top of that they put the chocolate ice cream and syrup. As I discovered, at that time in South Carolina they didn't like New Yorkers very much."

New Yorker Dan Blatt (army, Ft. Dix, 1962) was surprised to discover that all his sergeants were southerners with thick accents. "I went through two months of training and I swear, I could never understand a thing they were saying. The good news was that every second word they said was 'fuck,' because that was the only word I recognized."

By 1974, when Val Nicholas went through basic the situation had changed completely. "I'm African-American and my Drill Sergeant was an African-American. One night I was on fire watch and he was up late. He asked me to come into his office and started talking to me not as a Drill Sergeant but as a person. He talked about being black in the military and told me, 'You need to bear in mind what you do in the army doesn't just impact your life, but it's going to have an impact on what happens to all the other African-Americans working their way up behind you.'

"In basic we weren't black and white, we were all green. We had one kid who was barely educated and on Sundays he would come over to me with the comics and ask me to read them to him. At one point I offered to try to get him into a remedial reading class and he said to me, 'That's good for you because you're smart, but I'm not smart and that's why I like the army. I like that they tell me what to do and how to do it and when to do it. So I don't have to be the smartest guy to do it. So reading better is not something I'm looking to do.' That was a real education for me that people's goals are different, and you can't project your goal on anyone else."

A Memorable Reception:
The First Few Days

GENERAL CATLAY: I want to welcome you this morning to Fort Knox and the U.S. Army Training Center Armor . . . I think you're going to find that training here can be described as rigorous, probably also described as demanding, but you're going to find it's well within your capabilities. What we are going to try and do is give you the military training which, backed by your native instincts and native intelligence, is going to turn you into a soldier so that your reactions in times of stress are going to be a combination of instinct, native ability, and intelligence, reinforced by the military training that will give you the skills to react effectively.

—from the documentary *Basic Training,* by Fred Wiseman

THE SERGEANTS WHO PROCESSED us (those first few days) were mostly Vietnam veterans," Ben Currin (army, Ft. Bragg, 1968) remembers. "Their job was to make sure that we were in formation, that we showed up on time to eat, that we were at the right processing station at the right time, that we filled out all the necessary paperwork. They gave us a few preliminary tips about how to make a bunk, how to do a police call, how to pick up trash.

The first three or four days were relatively easy. But just when I began thinking, this isn't as tough as I heard it was, these guys showed up wearing Smokey the Bear hats. For someone like me, who had never been exposed to the military, I had no idea who they were. My first thought was that these guys must be forest rangers. Then they opened their mouths."

"I was seventeen years old when I joined the Marines, just out of high school," explains Tom Seaver (Marines, 1962, San Diego). "I had no idea what to expect when I showed up. Within the first few minutes I was standing on a set of yellow footprints and this crazed person was inches away from my face and screaming at me as loudly as possible—and I hadn't even done anything yet."

There is a rationale and a method behind the apparent chaos that greets a recruit when he or she arrives at basic training. In 1967 Peter B. Bourne wrote an article in *Psychiatry* entitled "Some Observations on the Psychosocial Phenomena Seen in Basic Training." "When a recruit arrives he is plunged into an alien environment, and is enveloped in a situation without relief. He is stunned, dazed, and frightened. The severity of shock is reflected in 17-hydroxycorticosteroid levels comparable to those in schizophrenic patients in incipient psychosis and which exceeds levels in other stressful situations. The recruit receives little, or erroneous information about what to expect, which tends to maintain his anxiety . . . Basic training is unique in American society."

On the first day of basic training "Everyone is starting from scratch," Joe Lisi points out. "Everyone has the same color toothbrush, same colored underwear, same haircut, everything is the same. It was done purposefully, I think, to eliminate any sense of individuality, so they can mold you into the young Marine they want you to be. It was done to bring everyone onto the same level as everyone else.

"Because you don't know how to march they tell you to line up asshole to belly button, 'Get in line, ladies, asshole to belly button,' as they marched us around to be issued gear, get our haircut and inoculations, towels, everything. We moved as a herd. I was so nervous that I was on Parris Island seven days before I had a bowel movement."

Because every member of a new recruit class starts even, the last thing anyone wants to do is attract attention by standing out from the group. Without any knowledge of the rest of the group, as Cindy McNally (air force, Lackland, 1975) learned, that can be a problem. "I was a doctor's daughter so I showed up for basic training in a little white pants suit," she remembers. "I didn't know any better. Nobody had told me anything about it but when I looked around and saw that everybody else was in bellbottoms and casual clothes I began to realize I'd made a mistake. When I got off the bus they got right in my face and said, 'This one's going to be a problem.' I hadn't said a word and they were already in my face."

Dan Blatt made a different mistake when he arrived at Ft. Dix in 1962. "I had brought a newspaper with me to read on the trip to the base. When I got off the bus I was carrying the *New York Times*. In retrospect that probably was a mistake. The sergeant took one look at that and immediately branded me 'A fucking New York Commie bastard.' A short time later we were taken over to get our uniforms. We just went through the line as people threw things at us. When I got an undershirt it looked like it was too small, so I stopped and politely asked the supply sergeant if they had anything in a large. Based on the response, I would have to say that was my second mistake."

"We arrived at the reception center in the pitch dark," Paul Satmaer (air force, Lackland, 1977) recalled. "We were standing on the exercise pad for about ten minutes when we heard this tapping coming closer. Tap, tap, tap. It was the metal taps on the shoes of our Training Instructors. They approached out of the darkness and then the booming started. First we played the game of picking up our suitcases and putting them down, picking them up and putting them down. I can't begin to describe how many times we did that. There was no logical reason for it, which was probably the reason for it. It was our introduction to military life. Then we were brought upstairs and told to take the first rack we came to. The beds were set in rows, side by side fifty to a squadron. Then we played the game of getting in and out of bed before the lights were turned off or turned on. The TI said, 'I'm gonna throw this switch and when it goes down I want you in bed before the lights go off and then I'm gonna flip it back on and I want you standing at attention before they go on.' We were literally trying to beat the speed of light. The most amazing thing was that they had us believing it was possible. Obviously it was a disaster; guys were falling down, getting hung up on the corner post of the bed; one recruit tried to leap into his bunk—and missed it, the bed, completely."

Take Everything Off the Top: Everything in the Military Is Uniform

"Excuse me, but is green the only color this comes in?"
—Goldie Hawn, getting her uniform in *Private Benjamin*

ANY CONNECTION A RECRUIT has with civilian life ends with the first military haircut. Actually, haircut probably is a misnomer because generally that word refers to some kind of styling. A military haircut is a crew cut, a total buzzcut, everything goes. It has been said that if it were any closer to the scalp it would have to be inside-out. The military haircut supposedly dates back to 1775, when George Washington ordered his troops to have their hair cut short to reduce the possibility of lice infection in camp. There is no speed record for a military haircut, but often months or years of perfectly grown and carefully groomed hair is completely gone in twenty to thirty seconds. Almost without exception, as military barbers will attest, as each platoon goes through the line at least one recruit will ask, "Would you take a little off the back, please." It is a well-known fact that military barbers are not known for their sense of humor. Female recruits do not have all their hair cut off; the only requirement is that they wear it above their collar and pulled back off the face, usually in some type of bun or pony tail. Tracy Harrell (air force, Lackland, 2000) remembers a group of female trainees who elected to have their hair cut short the third week of training because they realized that putting it up every morning took too much time and was too much trouble, but then the group got caught disobeying orders by leaving the salon and going for ice cream. "Our TI was furious and began talking about recycling them, sending them back to repeat several weeks of training. That night one of those girls was in the bathroom crying her eyes out. I mean she was hysterical, screaming and wailing, she was keeping everybody else awake. I was on guard duty and I tried to calm her down, telling her that the TI wasn't serious, nobody was going to be recycled. With tears rolling down her face she shook her head and said to me, 'That's not what's bothering me.' She pointed at her short hair. 'Look at this. My hair is so short now I'll never get married!' And then she started crying again."

When you get that haircut "You're not facing the mirror," Paul Setmaer explains. "When I sat down in the chair I had a full head of hair. Within seconds I felt a hot razor on my scalp. A few seconds later I was standing back up again. I remember turning around and looking in the mirror and not being able to find myself. I'd never seen myself that way. They were taking photographs for the cycle book and there's a picture of me with my hand on top of my head, leaning forward looking at the mirror with a strange expression on my face as if wondering, Oh my God. Is that me?"

Paul Steingruby III (army, Ft. Jackson/Ft. Benning, 1978) actually got two buzzcuts. "I never had long hair but I remember going into a room with three chairs. I recognized everyone in the line with me going in, but when we were through I didn't recognize anyone. They gave us a crew cut. I brushed my hand through it and thought, wow, they couldn't possibly cut it any shorter. It turned out I was completely wrong about that. That was my first lesson about the army. Three days later they marched us back in and buzzed it down to the skin."

During those first few days recruits also receive their inoculations. As far back as 1775 soldiers were being given a smallpox vaccine, while at present they receive a full spectrum of shots ranging from anthrax to yellow fever. "You stood in line and rolled up both sleeves," explains Mike LaRoche (army, Ft. Benning, 2004). "There were medics on either side of you. My memory is they were using pneumatic needles. As you walked through they just kept jabbing you. Pop, pop, pop, pop. You don't talk to anybody, you barely slow down to get a shot. My arms were sore but the last shot they gave us was a booster of some type right in the ass. Those shots in the arm were no more painful than someone punching you, and within a few hours I didn't even feel them, but that shot in the butt was the one that really hurt. It hurt going in and it burned. They ordered us to rub the hell out of it because if we didn't it would be sore for the next few days. First people came out of the barber shop rubbing their head, then after getting their shots they came out rubbing their butt. Everybody was standing around rubbing and squeezing, and days later, people were still gimping around."

"We had medics just jabbing us," says Dan Blatt. "As I went through I asked one of them, 'Have you done this before, Pal?'

"'Sure have,' he said, raising the needle high and aiming at my arm.

"'Don't you fucking miss,' I warned him.

"I don't think he liked that. As he punched the needle into my arm he said, 'I haven't missed in . . . ah shit!'"

During the few days spent at the reception station recruits move rapidly from area to area, learning rudimentary military skills, beginning with standing at attention. Attention is usually the first command a recruit is taught. As Kihm Winship (air force, Lack-land, 1968) says, "Heels together, toes slightly out, back straight, shoulders straight, thumb and forefinger touching pant seam, eyes ahead, no motion, no sound, staring at the back of the head of the man in front of you.

"Our Training Instructor was very specific, 'You will not move while at the position of attention. There will be no picking of the nose while at the position of attention.' Ah, I thought, a little humor, this won't be so bad."

The most difficult place at which to stand at attention has to be Parris Island. "Rather than mosquitoes we had sand fleas," remembers James Lambert (Marines, Parris Island, 1969). The sand fleas of Parris Island are legendary. They attack in waves, and among the first rules taught to recruits at Parris Island is you do not kill a sand flea. Sand fleas do not belong to recruits. Lambert continued, "The sand fleas were much worse than mosquitoes when it came to biting. When we were in formation at attention we had to learn to just ignore them. That was really hard. We weren't allowed to smack them, the Drill Instructors were really specific about that. When we were in formation and there was one on you, you had to learn how to look around without being seen looking around to see who was nearby, then make your move when nobody was looking. If you got caught smacking one you had to bury it. We had to dig a little grave and put it in there."

The tradition of the sand flea burial is an old one, and it first gained recognition in the 1957 classic movie *The D.I.*, in which Jack Webb created the unforgettable character of Marine Drill Instructor Gunnery Sergeant Jim Moore. With his recruit platoon standing rigidly at attention Sgt. Moore tells them, "You people are making me very unhappy. Just because the sand fleas get in your noses and your ears and crawl down your necks, you clowns think you have the right to kill them. I don't care how much they bite. You will pretend that you do not feel it . . . You can slap a sand flea in the jungle, if the enemy sees you move or hears you slap, you will be dead before you get your hand down. All your enemy needs is for you to slap a sand flea . . . (Pauses, and addresses a recruit) After I gave the orders you slapped a sand flea, didn't you?"

"Yes, Sir."

"You killed that sand flea, didn't you?"

"Yes, Sir."

"You murdered that poor little sand flea after I told you to let it eat all that it wanted to."

"Yes, Sir."

"If we would have been in combat yesterday, you would have gave away the whole platoon. We would all be dead just because of you, wouldn't we?"

"Yes, Sir. I'm sorry, Sir."

"Sorry? A dead Marine is never sorry, a dead Marine is just dead . . . Private Owens disobeyed orders and killed a sand flea. After chow this evening this whole platoon will fall out for burial detail. You will fall out with full packs, blankets, rifles, belts, bayonets, and canteens. You will find that flea that Private Owens murdered. You will find that exact same sand flea and you will bury it. Do you hear me?"

The sight of recruits standing in formation with blood running down their cheeks is not unusual. As Tommy Kilbride (Marines, Parris Island, 1980) says proudly, "PT [physical training] is PT, when you get to the end you're in such great shape it doesn't bother you anymore. But sand fleas can never be overcome. They're brutal, by May they're crawling all over your nose and in your ears, that's probably the most torturous part of training. But you get good at ignoring them. At the beginning you think they're going to drive you crazy, but eventually you develop such a strong sense of discipline you learn to ignore them. A mosquito could bite me for an hour now and if I chose to I wouldn't even smack it. That is discipline, and once you get it, you carry it with you throughout your life. If I choose not to be bothered by something physical, then so be it."

As Dennis Stead (Marines, Parris Island, 1960) learned, it wasn't only sand fleas and mosquitoes that made life so difficult. "I had a DI who did not like me at all. One day as the rest of my platoon was taking a break from the heat he called me out. He brought me over to the side where there were two other DIs from other platoons. At that time they would harass their own recruits to show other DIs how tough they were. This time he decided to pick on me. But as I stood there at attention the strangest thing happened; all of a sudden I felt this sharp pain in my right leg. I didn't move, I didn't say anything, I didn't respond in any way, but the pain got worse and worse. It turned out that a giant horsefly had landed on my leg and was drilling a hole so deep that blood began running down my leg. My sock was getting all bloody.

"My DI finally noticed that and asked, 'That hurt, Private Stead?'

"'No, Sir!' I said.

"He told me I could look, but warned me, 'Don't you move. If you move, you're dead.'

"I didn't move. I thought, no matter how much it hurts I am not moving. That damn fly kept drilling and the pain got worse. Those DIs actually made a bet on whether or not I would move—and of course my DI bet against me, that I would give up. I stood there and I took it, and I learned something about myself. I didn't move. After that, this DI treated me differently, he never picked on me again."

DI Does Not Stand for Devil Incarnate: The Men and Women Who Are King

"It was shortly after meeting drill instructor Fitch that I realized joining the Marine Corps might have been a bad decision."

—Jake Gyllenhaal as Anthony Swofford in *Jarhead*

Drill Sergeants are highly educated, qualified noncommissioned officers and the primary instructors in Initial Entry Training. They embody Army Values and are dedicated to training Soldiers to be strong defenders of the U.S. Army. Drill Sergeants lead by example.

—*The Soldier's Blue Book*, 2010

I will train them to the best of my ability. I will develop them into smartly disciplined, physically fit, basically trained Marines, thoroughly indoctrinated in love of corps and country." Or, as it has been interpreted, "Be damned sure no man's ghost returns to ask if your training programming had only done its job.

—*The Marine Drill Instructor's Creed*

I SPENT TEN DAYS in the reception area," recalls Tom Mellor (army, Ft. Benning, 1999). "Then they picked us up in a cattle car, a trailer with a big side door, and brought us down range. That was when basic training really began. When we got off that cattle car what's called the shark attack began. The Drill Sergeants came at us screaming. Right then I thought, okay, I'm in it now. It's over for me. Eventually the Drill Sergeants gave us their own speech, which was basically welcome to the infantry. You're here to learn how to kill. Nothing you learn here is going to help you in the real world. From this point on, killing is your day job."

After going through zero week at Ft. Jackson, Paul Steingruby III was shipped to Ft. Benning to begin basic. "What you see in the movies about recruits arriving in basic training and being attacked by Drill Sergeants, that's pretty accurate. The bus pulled in about 3:00 A.M. and this guy got on the bus and started cussing and calling us all kinds of names and told us we had thirty seconds to get off his bus and stand in formation. And we didn't even know what a formation was.

"He started blowing his whistle and people started scrambling over seats trying to find their duffel bags. That was impossible in the dark so they grabbed any bag and dragged it off with them. Eventually we were standing in a formation and we were all saluting the flag with our right hands, all of us except this one guy from Tennessee who was saluting it with his left hand. I looked over and the Drill Instructor was steaming, in the morning chill it literally looked like steam coming out of his ears. He practically leaped on this guy and demanded what the hell he was doing saluting with his left hand and the recruit explained that he had no choice, because 'I had my cigarette in my right hand.'

"That night he was introduced to the duck walk, and he spent the rest of the night duck walking around the building."

Brian Dennehy explains, "When a platoon is put together they assign you to a barracks and then three to five Drill Instructors come bursting through the door shouting contradictory orders. The point is to put you in a state of shock where you stay to some extent until the pressure eases off."

Mike LaRoche's platoon marched from Ft. Benning's reception area to their barracks, while their duffel bags and their civilian suitcases were trucked down and dropped in two huge piles about two hundred yards apart. "When we got there we were lined up about three hundred yards from the two piles. They had us line up in single file in eight columns. When they read off your social security number you were supposed to sprint toward either one of the piles to get your bags. You start sprinting but you don't know what you're doing. My only thought was I've got to get my bags, but as you start running the Drill Sergeants run with you and start slamming into you. They start demanding, 'What do you think you're doing?' The answer is you don't know what the right answer is. I didn't know how to answer but it didn't matter. I kept telling them, 'I have to get my bags.' What I eventually found out was that there is no right answer. Every answer is the wrong one. The point was to harass you, to break your wind.

"The whole time they kept dropping me, 'Do ten, do ten,' ten push-ups, then get up and keep running. When I got to the pile I had three or four seconds to find my bag. It was impossible, it was somewhere in a mountain of bags. So I had to turn around and run back until my number was called again. I didn't find my bag until the pile got whittled down. I don't have any idea how many hours it took because that was part of the objective. The army didn't want me to live on my time anymore, they wanted me to live on army time so they put me in time constraints that were impossible to meet. They actually gave me no time at all. There was no way I could find my bag in four seconds, but somehow I thought it was possible."

Michael Shapiro (army, Ft. Dix, 1959) witnessed what is arguably the worst introduction to basic training it is possible to imagine. "We were all reservists so we had a real attitude. I can remember getting on a bus and being driven from reception to our company area. When we got there the Drill Instructors started banging on the bus with their sticks to shake us up. As we got off the bus they kept it up. As one recruit got off the bus a sergeant hit him on the top of his helmet liner with a club. That recruit didn't hesitate. He turned around and decked that sergeant. I remember thinking, boy, that probably isn't the best way to get started."

"I served as an instructor for six years, two months, fifteen days," explained Mike Harrell (air force, Lackland, 1961). "My goal from the first day was to make them hate my guts." "I wanted them to hate me, I did everything I could to make them hate me. The reason why is they were all coming from different backgrounds, different religious, economic, and social backgrounds. I figured if I could give them a common enemy for the first few weeks, they would band together and learn how to work together. They had little or no self-discipline, so I had to impose discipline until they learned self-discipline. Their attitude became the only way we can get this guy off our backs is to work together. Slowly and surely they started working together and when I saw them coming together I would ease off. When they started getting things done without me yelling at them I didn't need to be so hard."

According to Master Instructor Joe "Tuffy" Tofuri, author of *Tuffy's Heroes,* and an air force TI for almost fifteen years, instructors had their own strategy for introducing recruits to the military. "This was something we would often do in the 1960s at Lackland when we picked up a new flight: At that time, most flights were composed of people from the same area of the country. We knew from experience that we would have the most discipline problems with flights coming from the east coast. There were always a few people in those groups with a negative attitude, Elvis wannabes and James Dean wannabes. This was during the Vietnam War, and we had to get these troops prepared to go to war. We didn't have time to deal with attitude problems. So we worked out a plan for an immediate and abrupt attitude adjustment.

"We would get someone, usually a young TI we trusted, to role-play the part of a new arrival for us. This plant would dress in civvies, and take his place in a new flight of 'rainbows.' New recruits are called rainbows because they're dressed in civilian clothes, which are all the colors of a rainbow. One time, I remember, I recruited a new Instructor for this job, explaining to him that I was going to do him the favor of allowing him 'to get your ass whooped tonight.' At first he didn't think it was much of a favor.

"Then I explained the plan to him. On the first night of every flight we had a mandatory incoming briefing. I told him, 'When we start briefing the flight every once in a while you snicker or make some wise-ass remark. One of us is going to chew your ass, and when we walk away you go ahead and tell us to go fuck ourselves or something like that. Act like a real hard ass. That's when we get to throw you down the barracks stairs.'

"That's what we would do. After our plant established himself as a wise-guy, we would literally grab him by his shirt, yank him off his foot locker, kick his ass down the hallway, and throw him down the stairway.

"Of course, the rainbows couldn't see that there was someone waiting halfway down the stairs to catch him. But the two of them would make enough of screaming racket to convince the recruits that we were serious. The recruits were stunned. And believe me, the point was emphasized when they never saw that 'recruit' again.

"It worked unbelievably well. We'd come back into the room,

and those trainees would be sitting on their footlockers like they had 2 × 4s nailed to their back. Their eyes were bulging. I mean, they were motivated. If they didn't know before, they knew now they were in a different world."

The relationship between a drill instructor and a recruit has been compared to a master and a slave but that's probably inaccurate. It's much worse than that. It's an often difficult and always complicated relationship in which these instructors have eight weeks to teach recruits an entirely new way of approaching life. The army calls them Drill Sergeants, the Marines refer to them as Drill Instructors, in the air force they are Training Instructors, and in the navy they are Recruit Division Commanders, but for the length of recruit training they are simply the all-powerful being. They have absolute power twenty-four hours a day, seven days a week, over the life of every member of their company. All the power of the military is invested in each one of them. Joe Russo (army, Ft. Leonard Wood, 1959) summed it up when he pointed out, "Sometimes it seemed like the whole United States Army was run by the same sergeant."

"They weren't out to impress you," Tom Jones emphasized. "They were out to change you from the person you were when you came in to the soldier they wanted you to be when you left."

Hal Fritz (army, Ft. Knox, 1966) describes his Drill Sergeant as "the personification of what you would expect to see in a Drill Sergeant; a small, wiry guy with tattoos on his arm. He was wearing the Smokey the Bear hat, a combat infantryman's badge on his uniform, and a cigarette hanging out of his mouth. He was as tough as nails, always on edge like he was sitting on razor blades, but he was always professional. He worked effortlessly day and night, whatever we were doing he was with us. When we marched in the rain he marched with us, when we had night duty, he was with us, always reminding us, 'You work as a team, you guys are going to be good.' He made us work as a team, always reminding us that when we were in combat our lives would depend on the people to our right and left. He encouraged those who had potential to be better and helped those who needed assistance. He told me I had potential, and if I wanted to stay in the army I could have a good career." Fritz later received the Congressional Medal of Honor for his heroic actions in Vietnam.

The most difficult problem Thomas Burke (army, Ft. Benning, 2004) had was not laughing when his Drill Sergeant lost his temper. "He was only about five feet tall and he would literally carry a small step stool around with him, and when he got mad at someone he'd put the stool down in front of that person and climb up so he could look them right in the eyes. He was a good teacher, but when he climbed up on his stool it was hard to take him seriously."

Instructors speak a unique and often colorful language. General George Washington wrote in a message to his commanders in 1776, "The General is sorry to be informed that the foolish and wicked practice of profane cursing and swearing . . . is growing into fashion; he hopes that officers will, by example as well as influence, endeavor to check it. . . . It is a vice so mean and low, without any temptation, that every man of sense and character detests it and despises it."

It would be accurate to report that Washington's admonition did not catch on. Or, as one legendary Drill Sergeant warned a recruit, "Unfuck yourself, Private, before I unfuck you."

As every recruit will attest, few men or women are better at the creative, colorful, and often hysterically funny use of the language than instructors. Among the legendary remarks: "What is your major malfunction, Private? You make the Rain Man look like a fucking genius!"

"Private, you are more fucked up than a football bat!"

"Now, I'm pissed. P-I-S-T, pissed!"

"I know I said it, Private. You know how I know I said it? Because I was there when I said it."

"If I tell you Christmas isn't coming, you do not put up a fucking tree."

When a recruit asked her Drill Sergeant to speak louder, he responded, "Can't you just listen harder?"

"You want to act the fool, Private, we will act the fool. And at the end there will be only one fool and that will be me!"

Female instructors can be just as profane as their male counterparts, for example the instructor who warned her platoon, "I'm gonna make you do side straddle hops until your Fallopian tubes fall out."

Future TI Mike Harrell went through his own basic with a trainee who just couldn't stay in step. Finally his TI exploded, warning him, "Private, if you don't get in step, I'm gonna knock you upside the head so hard that you will fart the Star-Spangled Banner backwards."

The army's 2009 Drill Sergeant of the Year, Michael Johnson (army, Ft. Benning, 2001), admits, "There were times I heard words coming out of my mouth and even I had to wonder where they were coming from. We're not supposed to address a trainee as anything but private, their last name and rank, or warrior. But the reality is that everybody does it. Sometimes you just think about the first two words that come together, just to get their attention. For example, when I was in basic a Drill Sergeant got so angry, so upset, he called somebody, 'cock smoke.' Cock smoke! That's an amazing combination of words. It doesn't mean anything at all. But so what? I thought, holy crap, I never heard anything like that."

There are Drill Sergeants with a sense of humor. Ben Currin

(army, Ft. Bragg, 1968) reports, "We had one guy who was short and thick and built like a tank, so our Drill Sergeant gave him the nickname Tank. We had another fellow with a round face who sort of resembled a Huey helicopter. We'd be in formation and our sergeant would say, 'Where is my tank?' Tank would put one arm straight out in front of him with his fist balled up, like the artillery barrel on a tank and come running out of the formation. Then our sergeant would call out, 'Where's my helicopter?' and that recruit would come out jumping on one foot, one hand spinning in circles over his head. Those two would be circling each other and when the sergeant ordered, 'Tank, shoot down that helicopter,' Tank would begin shouting 'Boom! Boom! Boom!' while Helicopter was going ta-ta-ta-ta. Whichever one got shot had to hit the ground, while all the rest of us were just cracking up."

Let's Definitely *Not* Get Physical

WHILE BASIC TRAINING INVOLVES a substantial dose of physical conditioning and discipline, instructors have never been permitted to physically abuse trainees, but it has happened. As Tom Bartlett (Marines, Parris Island, 1952) wrote in the magazine *Leatherneck,* "I remember being thumped on the gourd (hit on the head) and for two days I had a size 10 ½ double-E boot imprinted on the soft flap of my posterior." In some instances instructors literally ask permission from their platoons at the beginning of the cycle to be as tough as possible, suggesting that there are two ways of going through training, the soft way or the physical way, which theoretically toughens them up for combat.

While the Marine Corps takes great pride in being the toughest service, and its training is more physically demanding than that of the other services, Marine Corps training was fundamentally changed in April 1956 after six recruits drowned in Ribbon Creek during a night march through the swamps of Parris Island. Since that time Marine Corps rules prohibit instructors from touching recruits except in specific teaching situations. The other services also restrict instructors from physically abusing trainees—although the reality is that on occasion it still takes place.

"In the beginning I was really afraid for my life," remembers Dan Bierbaro (Marines, Parris Island, 1966). "They were brutal. I remember thinking, what have I done? I have to get out of here. They would get physical. I got ticked off at the sergeant because he punched me and I almost punched him back. Instead I looked him in the eye and he knew that if he crossed that line one more time I'd kill him. He didn't bother me again, but there were other kids who didn't stand up to him."

"Their job was to scare the living hell out of you," Dennis Stead (Marines, Parris Island, 1960) says, "and they did. This was only four years after those recruits drowned so everybody was very careful about everything they did. One night in the barracks the drill instructors took us aside and told us, 'Boys, we got two ways to go here. You can go one way or you can go the Marine Corps way. The Marine Corps way is we might beat the hell out of you, but we won't set you back. The other way is we won't touch you but you're going to be set back every time you screw up.' Getting set back meant you were sent to a platoon behind you, which added about two weeks to your time in basic. We all agreed we were going to do it the Marine Corps way, which meant we would take everything they dealt without complaining and without reporting them."

There was an acceptable reason for the physical abuse, Joe Lisi explains. When he was at Parris Island in 1969, "There was a kid from a small town in Alabama. When we were in class they would tell you that if you felt yourself starting to fall asleep stand up and lean against a wall. It was a hot, humid day and this kid fell asleep. The Drill Instructors saw him and all three of them pounced on him and knocked him out cold. I thought they'd killed him, but when he came back to consciousness they were so angry at him for being knocked out that they beat him again. They were all Vietnam veterans and they told us that people who didn't pay attention out there not only got themselves killed, but they got other Marines killed. This was serious business.

"We had one kid who was a real wise ass. One night the instructors tuned him up. They beat the crap out of him. He wrote to his congressman, which led to an investigation. Our instructors were relieved and we were given a new team. There was a second investigation and we were all questioned. When I was asked what I saw I told them. 'Nothing.' Then they asked me how that was possible because my bunk was right next to this kid's. I said, 'I was at attention and at attention the eyes and head are straight forward.' That was the end of it."

Physical punishment wasn't limited to the Marines. "We had a master chief in charge of our platoon," recalls Robert Oxford (navy, Great Lakes, 1966). "We had eighty-eight men from all over the United States. The chief was a pretty tough guy. When you had to talk to him you had to get down on the concrete floor on your toes and elbows. And if you let your stomach hit the floor he would kick you in the stomach. I can still remember the pain in my toes and elbows trying to hold my weight up for an extended period of time. I felt that he just enjoyed that torture. It happened every single day and I can remember going down and getting kicked in the stomach. I looked up at him with hate in my eyes and he said to me, 'That's good. Hate keeps a man alive.'"

In 1980, according to Thomas Kilbride, "It was commonplace. You'd wake up in the morning, stand at attention on the red line that's on the deck in front of your rack. If the Drill Instructor so decided he'd come in front of you and give you a bolt, a punch from his hip to your chest. Today Marine Drill Instructors could get court-martialed for that, but in my personal opinion it just made you tougher. You got knocked down, you got back up. You got knocked down again, you got back up again. You got pissed off when it happened, you didn't deserve it, but it was something that happened that toughened you up."

By 1993, "The official policy at the time was no hitting," explains Brian Deever (Marines, Parris Island, 1993). "But did it happen? Yes. They'd punch you in the stomach; they'd knock the wind out of you. But they didn't hit you in the face and it wasn't a beating."

As Val Nicholas recalls, even without that agreement his army Drill Sergeant found a way around the rulebook, "He knew he couldn't hit us, so instead he would play basketball. We would have to stand at attention against the wall and he would walk back and forth dribbling his basketball. When he wanted to make his point he would stop in front of a person and talk about how badly they had screwed up—and then toss the ball at their mid-section. It was a great incentive not to screw-up."

For Robert Hannah (army, Ft. Benning, 2005), "At first our Drill Sergeants were pretty tough. They tried to instill in each of us a basic fear of them; you'd better listen or there will be consequences. They tried to drill into us discipline and cleanliness. At times it got pretty unreasonable, but at the same time you put a bunch of seventeen-to-nineteen-year-old young men together in a stressful situation they're going to act like children no matter what you do. It was basically the angry father approach. At the beginning we had a few incidents, there were people who didn't like to be yelled at, some people who cried because they missed home, I think we had one person threatened suicide. But by the end of the cycle our Drill Sergeants had opened up and it wasn't difficult at all. In fact, during the last week of basic, the guy I bunked with, who was from Texas, literally asked me if I would please punch him in the face. Just like that, 'Do me a favor, just give me one good punch in the face real hard.'

" 'Um, mind if I ask why?' He then explained that his wife was coming to our graduation and he wanted to convince her that basic training was tougher than it actually was, so he needed me to give him a black eye."

The impact that an instructor has on a trainee can change his or her life—as well as save it. Ben Currin (army, Ft. Bragg, 1968), who eventually became a Drill Sergeant, made a point the day he graduated from basic training to "find Drill Sergeant Benjamin and thank him for kicking our butts all over Ft. Bragg and turning us into somebody. The last thing I told him was that one of my goals was to emulate him. I wanted to have that 101st Airborne Division Combat badge on my right sleeve and one day I wanted to wear that Drill Sergeant hat."

The Military Marches on Its Feet, Always to the Cadence of a Rhythmic Beat

They say that in the army the chow is mighty fine,
Chicken jumped right off the table and started marking time.
O how I want to go, but they won't let me go,
Hooooome, ooooome, ooooome, HEY!
They say that in the army the coffee is mighty fine,
But it looks like muddy water and tastes like turpentine.
They say that in the army the money's mighty fine,
They give you hundred dollars and take back ninety-nine.

—Marching cadence

TRAINEES MARCH. THEY MARCH in formation from class to class, they march for fitness, they march for endurance. Armies have always marched. As Baron von Steuben wrote, "The march of columns is an operation so often repeated, and of so much consequence, that it must be considered as an essential article in the instruction of both officers and men. . . . The whole column must always begin to march, and halt, at the same time, and only by order of the commanding officer."

BASIC

When a basic combat trainee is learning to become a soldier he no longer walks—he marches. He marches over every type of terrain imaginable. . . . The objectives of this type of training are to teach the individual soldier the principles of march discipline, march hygiene, preparation and adjustment of packs, and to provide a series of practical exercise in cross-country marches. . . . Trainees test their training by experience and learn a final lesson: to cherish a most precious piece of equipment—their feet.

—Fort Bragg Training Center *Yearbook, January 1969*

Marching is the essential skill learned in basic training. During basic training recruits march, and they march with full gear for as long as twenty-five miles. When trainees are not marching, they're jogging. Or moving at "double-time." "It seemed like all we did was march," remembers Tony Vaccaro (army, Camp Van Dorn, Mississippi, 1943). "We started with five miles, the third week we did twenty miles, and by the end we did fifty miles."

There are many problems trainees will face during basic. The large number of them have never been away from home for an extended period, and many will get homesick. Drill Instructors have to deal with an endless variety of their charges' personal problems— death in the family, tornado destroyed the farmhouse and barn, girlfriend pregnant by best friend. Put young Americans into a military unit, and they will generate no end of personal problems, real and imagined, and each requires handling in one way or another. The DI, with the responsibility of training troops, must balance his mission with the requisite amount of compassion.

But few of the difficulties that arise are more painful than blisters. The combination of new boots and long marches almost inevitably leads to large, liquid-filled eruptions at the most irritable places on the foot and ankle. Of course, blisters in basic training aren't painful—so long as they happen to somebody else. No matter how hard they try, most trainees will get blisters. Why are they so prevalent? Because trainees march, and they march a great deal.

There is only one guaranteed effective treatment for blisters: Don't get blisters. Anthony Shaffer (army, Ft. Gordon, 1981) discovered an important secret for preventing them: "We used nylon knee-high socks to shine our boots, but they were also great on road marches. We found out that if you wore nylons under your wool socks, you could avoid getting blisters because the nylons absorbed the sweat better than wool. We'd wear them under the issue wool socks and we would never get blisters." It also has been reported that pantyhose work equally well—although the risk to a male trainee of being caught with pairs of pantyhose in his foot locker probably outweighs the reward.

Baron von Steuben emphasized the importance of marching in his drill manual, writing, "The greatest attention on the part of the officers is necessary at all times, but more particularly on a march: The soldiers being then permitted to march at their ease, with the ranks and files open, without the greatest care, these get confounded one with another; and if suddenly attacked, instead of being able to form immediately into order of battle, the whole line is thrown into the utmost confusion."

The term used by von Steuben, "ranks and files," has come to mean common people, but it actually was a military phrase, the ranks meaning those people marching abreast or next to each other and the files being in front and behind.

Marching in step builds teamwork, cohesion, and unit discipline. Among the very first things every trainee is taught is how to stay in step with their platoon, meaning that everybody is stepping forward with the same foot at the same time. What could possibly be any easier? There was one member of Paul Steingruby III's platoon who simply "could never march right. He was always out of stride with everybody else. Our Drill Sergeant tried everything to get him in step, but nothing worked. Finally he found a very practical solution to that problem: He ordered everybody else to get in step with him."

It is, perhaps, in the endeavor of marching that the inherent humanity and pragmatism of Drill Instructors bubble reluctantly to the surface. There is nothing more infuriating than being unable, through any means, to get troops to do something they cannot do. This puts the onus on the DI, someone whose demeanor is normally a vehicle for coercion, to find creative solutions.

Tracy Harwell had a typical problem trainee in her air force flight, explaining, "When you move your right leg your left arm is supposed to naturally move forward, and when you step with your left leg your right arm goes forward. But we had a trainee whose body didn't move that way. His body was out of sync. There was nothing our TI could do about that, so every time we had a drill inspection he was assigned to dorm guard duty." Of course, there is the argument that anyone who is too uncoordinated to walk has no business on guard duty, but in almost every unit in history, when the unit went to the field, left behind to guard the barracks were the organization's most inscrutably inept knuckleheads.

Norman Batansky (army, Ft. Jackson, 1969) admittedly was "a slow runner and my stamina wasn't great, so these marches were hard for me. I was always near the back of the pack, and one day our Drill Sergeant ordered, 'Batansky, fall out.'

"I told him, 'No, Sarge, I can do this.' But he repeated his order for me to fall out. I did but then I wondered, 'I can make it. Why did you want me to do that?'

"And he said, ' 'Cause I want somebody to talk to while we're walking along.' A Drill Sergeant with a heart."

The marching commands are reasonably basic: Forward march, right face, left face, and about face. About face, or "wheeling," as it once was known, can be the most difficult for a recruit to master, and almost inevitably at least one soldier will trip over his own feet and spin awkwardly onto the ground. Val Nicholas was given the honor by his Drill Sergeant of marching his platoon from one station to the next. You have to be able to count cadence, and to be able to distinguish left from right, neither of which is particularly difficult. Being in charge, as we all discover, carries with it not only the prestige of authority but also the burden of responsibility. And when you are a recruit and not yet skilled, that burden can be very heavy indeed.

"I was learning to march with my troops," Nicholas recalls, "and I couldn't figure out which foot to turn them on. As I watched in complete horror I marched them right into the side of the mess hall, where they piled up onto each other. I saw it happening, and it was so unbelievable there wasn't anything I could do to stop it. At that moment I couldn't remember the commands. And they listened to me: They just kept marching right into that wall like it was some terrible movie.

"The first thought that popped into my mind was the number of push-ups the Drill Sergeant was going to make me do. It was worse than that: all the garbage and grease was thrown into a trench near the mess hall—and I had to do those push-ups directly over that trench. Neither the memory of those people walking right into the wall nor the smell of that trench has ever gone away."

"When we set out at 6:00 in the morning for a fifteen-mile march, it was already 100 degrees," recalled David Fisher (army, Ft. Leonard

Wood, 1969). "I was in one of the last platoons, and part of the march went through an area under construction. All the vegetation had been removed, leaving just light brown dirt. It had rained the night before and as we came over a hill I could see way in the distance a huge mud puddle, and as each soldier walked by he was dipping his helmet into this water and pouring it over his head. I remember thinking, there is no way I'm gonna pour that filthy water over my head, but by the time we reached the hole the water was gone and all that was left was mud. I didn't even hesitate. I scooped up as much mud as possible in my steel pot and put it on my head, and just felt that unbelievably cool mud dripping down my face."

Working together as a unit, even if it is on a task as prosaic as marching, is like many other team endeavors: It has a unifying effect, and it imparts the strength of the unit, the strength of many, can be the individual. As onerous and unpleasant as it to, marching demonstrates in a convincing way that the whole is greater than any one member, and for trainees, the last forced march is a rite of passage that stays with them forever.

"At Ft. Benning when we finished that fifteen-mile march they have a little ceremony," explains Matt Riker (army, Ft. Benning, 2005). "We did the march, and at the end, the entire company formed a huge circle and in the middle they had a big pot filled with what was called 'grog.' It looked really cool. There was smoke pouring out of it. It had cranberries and God knows what else in it. I'm sure at one time it had alcohol in it, but now it's just a big sugar high. Actually, it was pretty disgusting. They probably called it 'grog' because nobody really wanted to know what was in it. It didn't matter though, because after that hike it was delicious—although after that hike pretty much anything would have been delicious. As we stood around, our Drill Sergeants gave a great motivational speech congratulating us on becoming soldiers. Then everybody took their cups, dipped them in this pot, and toasted each other!"

For Shawn Herbella (army, Ft. Jackson, 2004) a fifteen-mile forced night march was the final task in basic. "We were out in the field for a week, and then we had to hike back carrying all our gear. By that time I had stress fractures in both my shins. It was really hard on my body just making it through that, but then in the middle of the night I came up over a hill, and they were all waiting there for us. There was patriotic music playing, flags were flying, and as we got to the end our Drill Sergeant was there to shake our hands. It was a very emotional moment for me. I made it."

Apparently there have always been trainees who have difficulty staying in step, or even knowing their right from their left. "There was always one person who couldn't get it," remembers Saul Wolfe (army, Ft. Dix, 1958). "We had a sergeant who would stand next to that person when we were marching screaming into his ear, 'Your left, your left,' and every time he did that the right foot would hit the ground. Finally, in desperation, he screamed, 'Your other left, stupid!'"

Although humans are specially constructed to walk upright—indeed it is one of the capabilities that distinguishes us from most other animals—there is a certain percentage of trainees who are incapable of the simple task of walking in step to the beat of a drum. During the American Revolution if a soldier was having difficulty staying in step, a piece of straw was affixed to one of his feet and some hay to the other one, and then the instructor would call out, "Hay-foot, straw-foot, hay-foot," and so on. Eventually, a more efficient solution, the cadence call, evolved. The cadence call is a responsive marching song that establishes a rhythm enabling all the troops to stay in step.

In its simplest and least creative form, a cadence call includes the words "left" and "right," so that even the least gifted trainee could get the point, "You had a good home when you *left*," which would immediately be answered in chorus by the marching platoon, "You're *right*."

INSTRUCTOR: The police were there when you *left*.
PLATOON: You're *right*.
INSTRUCTOR: Your girl was there when you *left*.
PLATOON: You're *right*.
INSTRUCTOR: Sound off . . .

Music has been part of military culture throughout American history. "Yankee Doodle Dandy" is a pre-Revolutionary British and American marching song, and during the Civil War troops would proudly sing "The Battle Hymn of the Republic" and "When Johnny Comes Marching Home" to raise their spirits. "When the Caissons Go Rolling Along" and "Over There" were sung by American troops as they marched into World War I and turned the tide in favor of the Allies. The navy's "Anchors Aweigh" was written in 1906, reportedly as a tribute to the U.S. Naval Academy Class of 1907. "From the Halls of Montezuma" became the official Marine Corps hymn in 1929, and "Off We Go Into the Wild Blue Yonder" was the award-winning entry in a 1938 magazine contest to write an official Army Air Corps song.

None of these marching songs involved a cadence count. According to legend, the military cadence count was born at Ft. Slocum, New York, in 1944 when an African American soldier named Willie Duckworth began calling out "Sound-off 1-2, sound off 3-4; Cadence count 1-2-3-4, 1-2! 3-4!" and that was picked up by the other soldiers marching in his formation. The catchy call appeared to put a spring in the steps of the marchers and was quickly adopted by other units. The "Duckworth Chant" spread rapidly throughout the military and is still a staple of marching today.

Irwin Hunter remembers watching the segregated black troops marching to their own rhythm at the Naval Training Station Sampson, in Lake Seneca, New York in 1944. "All the blacks in the navy were training to be steward's mates, kitchen duty. We had no contact with them; at that time the military was very segregated. But I remember how the black boots attracted everybody's attention whenever they marched because of the way they sang to keep in rhythm. That was something different."

The original World War II cadences focused on subjects universal to soldiers: "What the hell are we doing here? Let's go out and have a beer." But new cadences have been written for each American military involvement. Korean War trainees sang, "I don't know but I've been told, North Korean girls are mighty cold." Those people who served during Vietnam will remember a cadence designed around the tune of the Coasters' "Poison Ivy," "Late at night when you're sleeping, Charlie Cong comes a-creeping all a-roun-n-n-d. Vietnam!" Most recently troops headed for Iraq and Afghanistan sounded off, "When you get there this is what you'll do, You gotta kill Al-Qaeda for me and for you; We got to get them back for what was done, On September 11, two-thousand-one."

There are no official regulations governing cadence calls and in fact all of them are created by instructors and trainees and generally reflect contemporary culture. When Kevin Robert Meade (army, Ft. Leonard Wood, 1987) was a Drill Sergeant in 2002 he recalls, "I liked to have stuff come off the top of my head and just roll with it. As long as it rhymed and the troops were running with me I was happy. One, for example:

I don't know, but I think I might; hit the clubs come Friday
   night,
With baggy pants and shiney shoes, tell you what I'm
   gonna do;
Slide to the left, slide to the right; Electric glide on a Friday
   night.
I'll look up and who do I see; Britney Spears trying to get
   with me.
Britney Spears I love her so, I stay up late to watch her video.

As Peter Flood (army, Ft. Dix, 1968) explains, "We had an in-structor we really liked. So in his honor we created a cadence call, 'We're the men of F Platoon, the rappers of the night; We're Ser-geant Caso's raiders, we'd rather fuck than fight.' Maybe some of the other sergeants didn't like it, but Sergeant Caso loved it!" Both Flood and Caso would be disappointed to learn that, when soldiers sang a similar cadence in the 1960s, it was already a generation old. When the military services were almost exclusively male, as expected, the cadence calls were politically incorrect. "Got a gal lives on a hill; She won't do it but her sister will." While an element of political correct-ness has snuck into cadences in the last decade, there is a seemingly unending list of cadences referring, in the most explicit and often unpleasant ways, to genitalia, sexual acts, and various nationalities.

In fact, what is arguably the best known cadence tells the entire story of a relationship, "The prettiest girl, I ever saw, was sipping whisky right through a straw; I picked her up, I laid her down, her long blond hair lay on the ground; The wedding was a formal one, her father had a big shot gun; And now I've got a mother-in-law, and fourteen kids who call me Pa!"

Which, of course, was similar to another classic, "Left my wife in New Orleans, with forty-eight kids and a can of beans."

While most cadence calls are quickly, and thankfully, forgotten, there are several that have been passed down through the generations. Gene DeSantis (army, Ft. Jackson, 1966) recalls several of them. "Once they get into your head they never leave. I remember as each platoon came jogging by they were calling or singing cadences like, 'I want to be an Airborne Ranger, I want to live a life of danger,' 'My girl's a talker, she's a New Yorker; She's got a pair of legs, just like two whisky kegs; She's got a head of hair, just like a grizzly bear; she's got a pair of hips, just like two battleships.' Probably the one everybody who ever went through basic sang, 'We are Delta, mighty mighty Delta; Everywhere we go, people wanna know; who we are.'" For anybody who has been there, it is literally impossible to read these words without hearing the tune or rhythm behind them.

Many popular cadence calls feature a mythical civilian named Jody, the man who stayed home when the soldier went to war and stole the trainee's girlfriend or wife, car, and possessions. Eventually though, as more women joined the military, Jody became the temptress at home making time with a husband or boyfriend. Jody was the universal SOB, capable of anything. Jody slept with your girlfriend, drove your car, spent your money, and even ate your mother's home cooking.

Nobody really knows Jody's origins, but he's become the Paul Bunyan of back-stabbers, the omnipresent draft-dodging sneak, homewrecker, seducer, and thief. Atlas held up the world; Jody stole your girl. In fact, Jody was so prevalent that cadences have even become known as "Jodies." Among the classic Jodies:

Ain't no use in looking down, there ain't no discharge on
   the ground;
Ain't no use in going home, Jody's got your girl and gone;

Ain't no use in feeling blue, Jody's got your sister, too;
Ain't no sense in looking back, Jody's got your Cadillac.
Your baby was lonely as can be, 'til Jody provided some
    company.

Finally, cadence calls are also used to poke fun at the rival services, which is not surprising, since even at a time in which joint operations are highly valued, loyalty to your branch is rampant. "I don't know but I been told; navy wings are made of gold; I don't know, I've heard it said; air force wings are made of lead."

During basic or bootcamp trainees are not soldiers, sailors, airmen, or Marines, instead they are trainee, recruit, or private. For a time, the air force called its recruits "airman," and that proved to be a problem for Paul Ehrman (air force, Lackland, 1965). "Initially I went to Officer's Training School, but a few days before graduation I opted out, which shaved a year off my commitment. But because of my time in OTS I knew the air force manuals front cover to back cover, because we were tested on that material frequently. At one point after leaving Officer's Training, I was on a detail, and a first lieutenant walked passed me. I had this sticky stuff in my hands so I didn't salute. He stopped me and said, 'Don't you salute when you pass an officer?'

"I explained, 'I'm on a detail so I don't have to salute.'

"He didn't like that. 'Who told you that?'

"'Air Force Manual 30-15 states that when on detail the NCOIC in charge salutes for the entire detail.' Who knows, that might have been true, but one thing for sure, if it wasn't, this officer didn't know it. He asked me who was in charge of my detail. 'O'Hara,' I said, thinking of our company clerk, a friend of mine. This officer was getting angrier, so he asked for my name. I told him, 'Ehrman.'

"That wasn't good enough for him. 'I didn't ask for your rank, I asked you for your name.'

"'I know,' I told him. 'Ehrman.'

"'Airman, I'm going to give you one more chance. What is your name?'

"I tried again, 'Ehrman,' I said. Two days later O'Hara informed me I was to report immediately to the base commander's office. I figured, this isn't good. My assumption was that the commander wanted to speak with me about dropping out of OTS, but I had no choice. I walked into his office and he was sitting behind his desk. He looked up at me and just stared for a few seconds without saying a word. 'You wanted to see me, Sir?' I said.

"He smiled. 'Not really,' he admitted. 'I just wanted to meet Airman Ehrman.'"

Everything Is Public for Privates

IN EACH SERVICE THE first few weeks are a whirl of activity designed to introduce each trainee to the rigorous demands of military life, with the objective being to completely change his or her view about how they fit into society. Before entering the service, each trainee took for granted a certain level of freedom. They were able to make individual choices—but basic training is a group activity. There is no individual freedom. The Marines, for example, do not allow trainees to use personal pronouns, and there is no such thing as privacy.

For some, this loss of individual liberty is a psychological shock that proves difficult or impossible to handle, but the service's intention is to mold the recruit into a member of a well-trained team able to perform his or her duties under all circumstances. Or, as the army describes it, "Showing the capability to operate effectively in a stressful environment."

"The first few days are designed to make sure you don't get enough sleep," remembers John Langeler (navy, Great Lakes, 1966). "Soon as we got there they threw us into an old barracks with ratty mattresses and no blankets in October and ordered us to get to sleep. Then the second everybody is asleep, they turned on the lights and marched us off to eat. I was so totally exhausted those first few days I couldn't even remember my name. I would have done anything just to get a couple of hours of sleep."

Everything most people are used to doing in private suddenly has to be done publicly. In most barracks the doors have been removed from the toilet stalls, the showers are communal, and there are as many as eighty people living and sleeping in a single barracks room. Joe Lisi admits, "The hardest part was getting used to the total lack of privacy. They had a row of heads, and each head is porcelain with a thick rim. There was no toilet seat. I was just so nervous I couldn't shit. So finally, that first Sunday I went to church and asked the chaplain for permission to make an emergency head call. That was the first privacy I'd had. I went in there and finally was able to go to the bathroom. Thank God—literally."

"My father always told me when I went into a public bathroom I should cover the toilet seat with toilet paper," explains Ira Berkow (army, Ft. Leonard Wood, 1958). "Then I went to basic. The bathroom had four toilets directly across from four other toilets; there was no separation, and so basically we would sit knee-to-knee. For the entire first week every one of us was constipated because we were too embarrassed, but after that nobody paid any attention to it. In fact we started having meetings in the toilet because it was a place we could have some privacy as a group.

"At first I did cover the seat with toilet paper, but we weren't given enough of it and everyone started bitching at me, so I tried to be a little more sparing. But maybe that was an important lesson I took away from basic training—I didn't have to cover the seat with toilet paper."

Robert Hanna (army, Ft. Benning, 2005) remembers being "shocked" to discover that "the latrines were not open like they were in other barracks. We had doors! Doors meant privacy. We all looked at those doors and immediately had one thought—what a perfect place to get some sleep during the day."

As John Langeler adds, at Great Lakes the navy made the bathroom situation just a little more difficult. "We had ten heads inside stalls and ten urinals. But when we woke up in the morning eight of those ten stalls and eight of the urinals would be roped off so we couldn't use them. Supposedly that was to emphasize that aboard ship water is rationed. It certainly taught most of us self-control."

There also is no such thing as a leisurely shower, and it doesn't matter that the service stresses the importance of cleanliness as a means to keep infection rare among large numbers of people living together in relatively primitive conditions. "During our first week in the training platoon we did what was called 'shower drills,'" explains Joshua Barnes (air force, Lackland, 2006). "We would strip naked at our bunks, get a bar of soap, and line up. We would then run from the bay into the showers. The shower heads were lined up along two walls, and we had to move steadily along those two walls. We were not permitted to slow down or stop under a shower head. Not that anyone wanted to; our TIs had turned every other shower either scalding hot or freezing cold. Basically, fifty-five men showered in less than five minutes, but it wasn't the showers that caused the real problem. The real problem was getting out of the shower.

"Three issues came together: Everybody wanted to get out of there as quickly as possible, the tiled floor was soaking wet, and we were all young men—meaning that above everything else the one thing we most wanted to avoid was touching anybody else's naked body. Imagine fifty-five naked freezing guys trying desperately not to slip on the tiles while avoiding each other—then running into each other in a huge jumble; naturally everybody fell. There was this huge pile-up of fifty-five naked trainees writhing on the floor trying desperately to move as quickly as possible without getting touched or touching anyone. The more people tried to avoid it, the worse it got. It was impossible, which I guess was the objective.

"By the time we got through that I think everybody had lost whatever inhibitions they might have had about dealing with other people."

Myth #1: The Saltpeter Solution

They feed us "Salt Peter" in our food. That's a certain chemical to keep you very unemotional.

—Pvt. Herbert Beyer, writing to his wife from the Army Air Force Basic Training Center in Miami Beach, Florida, 1943

PROBABLY THE MOST COMMON myth about basic training or boot camp is that the military secretly puts saltpeter, or potassium nitrate, in food to reduce the trainees' sexual drive. No one knows when this myth began circulating, but it may go back as far as World War I. Like many rumors that circulate among troops, there is no truth to it. Saltpeter, which is used in explosives, is not an antiaphrodisiac. Besides, the military already has a method of reducing trainees' sexual drive during basic training—it's called basic training. At the end of each day in boot camp a trainee is usually too tired and too stressed even to have a libido, let alone to think about what he would do with one.

"I guess like everybody else we heard the rumor that one of the shots we received had saltpeter, or that it was in our food," remembers Chad Davisson (Marines, San Diego, 1993). "Supposedly it was an attempt to reduce erections. We learned for sure that it was not true one cold morning when we were standing at attention right out of the rack. One recruit was standing stiff for all to see. It was pretty hard to miss it—and our instructors didn't miss anything. Once our Drill Instructor saw it, it was on. 'What is this?' he screamed and within seconds the recruit was completely surrounded by Drill Instructors. They were in his face and in his crotch, screaming at both of them. Meanwhile, the rest of us were trying desperately to hold tight and not lose it. Finally, one Drill Instructor took off his Smokey and hung it right on the little soldier. Then he warned the recruit, 'You keep that hanging right there. If my cover touches the deck you're a dead man!' At that point the rest of us were having trouble holding back our tears. The recruit was trying everything to hold up that hat. He arched his back, his eyes were riveted closed as he tried to focus, he was straining, but obviously it was impossible. Within a few seconds his salute went limp—and the cover fell to the floor.

"That was it, we lost it, we lost it out loud—and nobody cared that we had to spend the rest of the morning in the sand being thrashed."

The Biggest Cover-up: Making the Military Bed

THERE IS ONE SKILL that every person who has been through military basic training will retain forever: the ability to make a bed with hospital corners. Like throwing a hand grenade, it has limited application outside the military, but as trainees learn during their first week, there is only one correct way to make a bed—and that is any way other than the way you are doing it.

Making a bed according to strict standards is the military's way of teaching recruits how to pay attention to detail, but because of the Drill Instructors' numbing insistence on expertise, the ability to perform the task survives much longer than the lesson that it's the little things that always get you into trouble.

There are about as many individual steps in making a bed as in assembling a jet airliner, although making a bed to military standards is probably more complicated. Each step in making a bed must be executed perfectly, or else you can't do the ensuing steps properly, and folding hospital corners at exactly 45 degrees is a skill acquired after many hours of painstaking practice, encouraged by deafening, obnoxious, and profane assistance from a Drill Sergeant.

As a Fort Knox Drill Sergeant instructs trainees, "The first step is to take one sheet and place it on the rack from side-to-side. Line up the end of the sheet with the bottom of the mattress, making sure the overhang is equal. Next you want to kneel by the head end of the rack and tuck the sheet up under so it is flush. Next you want to go to one side of the head end of the mattress and start doing the 45 degree corner. You do that by lifting up the bottom end of the sheet and pulling it back so as to have the overhang pulled tightly, and tuck it underneath. Next you will let the excess form the 45 degree angle. You place your hand under to make it smooth and then you will tuck the excess under. You always want to make sure you smooth out the sheet; you continue tucking the excess sheet all the way down to the foot end of the rack. Next you will go to the other side and proceed in the same manner as the first side. Next you will want to take the second sheet and line it up with the head of the rack, making sure the overhang is equal on both sides.

"Next step you want to take the first green blanket and place it on the rack. That has U.S. stamped on it for United States. This should be readable when seen at the bottom of the rack. Place the blanket on the rack, just like the sheet, making sure there is an equal overhang on both sides of the rack. You want to line up the top of the green blanket approximately twelve inches from the head of the rack. Next you will start tucking the blanket in with the sheet, making sure that everything is smooth. Again do the 45 degree angle at the foot end of the mattress, making sure it is retained by folding up excess blanket, tucking it smooth underneath, placing your hand there, and bringing the excess part of the blanket all the way down. Next you will go to the other side and do the hospital corner or 45 degree angle you did on the other side until it is complete." Simple.

Actually, much to the dismay of some former DIs, the advent of fitted sheets has rendered these vital bed-making skills superfluous.

For trainees, of course, the drill of making a bed was merely the impetus to find creative ways to beat the system. Cindy McNally (air force, Lackland, 1975) reveals one of the common tricks, "If the hospital corners weren't exactly at 45 degrees the instructor ripped it up and you had to start again. So what we did to pull it tight was to lay the blanket over the bed and then get on the floor and crawl underneath. Then we pulled it tight through each one of those little springs."

Some instructors literally would bounce a quarter on a rack to test if it was tight enough. Norman Batansky had a better system: He would pay another recruit a quarter a day to make up his bunk, but only if it passed inspection. That may have been a much better deal than Richard Goldman made the first day of training. "I didn't know how to make a bed or shine my shoes," he says, "so I agreed to pay another trainee ten dollars a week to make my bed, shine my shoes, and keep everything up to date."

Obviously, given enough time it was possible to make a bed with hospital corners that would pass inspection, but there are only two times in the military: first, not enough, and second, hurry up and wait. When they awake, most trainees wonder: Is it still really late last night, or is it very early this morning? Generally the first sound every recruit hears in the morning was the tap-tap-tapping of their instructor coming into the barracks. "We all wore horseshoe taps on our boots and shoes for psychological reasons," admits DI Dan Blatt. "It enhanced our performance. I would get to my troops' barracks at four in the morning. They told me they would listen for me coming up the stairs, and they claimed they could tell what kind of mood I was in, meaning what kind of day they were in for, from the beat of my taps on the stairs."

At Lakeland in 1969, Kihm Winship remembers it took a mere five minutes to go from being in bed to being fully dressed and in perfect formation outside. "At exactly 5:00 A.M. our TI turned on the lights and screamed GEETTTTUPPPPP! We were up before he finished. I once saw a man sleep through a wake-up call; the sergeant pushed over his bunk, knocking over two other bunks. I had an upper bunk and one time I leaped out of bed and landed right on the guy in the lower bunk. We didn't have time to argue.

"Within seconds we pulled on our clothes, which had been left lying the night before in perfect order on top of our footlocker. The shirt was already buttoned, and so we just pulled it over our head; there was no time to button a shirt. We were dressed in thirty seconds, unless we had to lace up combat boots, in which case it would take a full minute. The second minute was spent making the bed. We learned to sleep without moving, our knees high, so we wouldn't have to remake the corners at the bottom. The bed would be perfect before the end of the second minute, and then we had one minute to clean our detail. You could throw in a run to the bathroom, but only if you were really in agony."

Like many others Steven Singer (army, Ft. Polk, 1970) discovered the most extreme solution to this problem. "Once my bed was made correctly, I just didn't crawl under the covers at night. I'd sleep on top and when I got up in the morning all I had to do was tighten the corners of the blankets."

Christine Knight (army, Ft. Sill, 2000) remembers running outside her barracks to get into formation at "O-dark-30. I'd spent so much time getting my bed in order that I was late getting outside for PT. As I ran outside I realized that I had forgotten to put my bra on. I have never been a small girl on top so this was going to be a problem. I told my Drill Sergeant that I needed to go back to the barracks. Naturally, she was sympathetic, she called over the other Drill Sergeants and told them, 'We have a hussy in here. This girl is walking around with no bra.'

"One of the other Drill Sergeants asked the company, 'Anybody else here need to put their bra on?' Thank goodness a couple of other women raised their hands. I wasn't the only one. I was thinking how dumb I was until the same sergeant asked the men, 'Any of you males forget to put on your drawers?'

"I was so satisfied when several men put up their hands—they had been in such a hurry they had forgotten to put on their underwear."

Reflections on the Military:
In Quest of the Perfect Shine

A MONG THE OTHER SKILLS that trainees acquire during basic that have limited use in civilian life is the art of shining boots. Really, really shining boots. "I excelled at spit-shining my boots," remembers Anthony Shaffer. "This is a subject that everybody has their own opinion about, there were a lot of techniques, but for me it was pressure and polish. I used standard Kiwi black polish, a little water, and rubbing in small twirls. The sergeant actually put his boots next to mine and said, 'I'm gonna remember you.' Then he wrote me a letter of commendation! My secret was that after my boots were shining I used nylon knee-highs to keep them buffed."

Brian Deever (Marines, Parris Island, 1993) believed that a quality spit shine required actual spit. "Other people would use tap water, I used spit. I always believed there was something about saliva that made your boots shine better."

Who knew there could be so many different methods of shining a boot? Some Marines would wipe down their boots with rubbing alcohol before applying polish, which would extend the life of the gloss. Later they would learn that applying a layer of pure beeswax serves as a great bottom coat. There were the shortcuts, of course;

admittedly many recruits found salvation in sponge or spray-on glossy polish. Among purists it generally was agreed that Kiwi provided the glossiest shine. Some people heated polish on the lid of the can into a pasty liquid before applying it, while others wet it. The biggest debate was what type of cloth to use for buffing. Among the popular choices were cotton balls, a white T-shirt, flannel gun patches, a jeweler's polishing cloth, handkerchiefs, and, especially in the Marines, cloth baby diapers. Followed by a rigorous buff with a fine-bristled brush.

The original shined black combat boots were introduced in 1957, replacing a modified brown service shoe to which a leather cuff had been added during World War II, and for almost fifty years provided Drill Sergeants with a good means to measure a trainee's commitment. "I grew up in an army where boots told the whole story of who you were," said Drill Sergeant of the Year 2004 Jason W. Maynard. "If they were shiny, then you were 'squared away.'"

In 2006 the army's traditional green battle dress uniform—which included highly-shined black boots—was replaced by a camouflaged combat uniform and more practical rough, tan-colored boots that did not need to be shined. Conditioned by a decade in Southwest Asia, the army assumed it would be spending a lot of time in desert environments and changed the uniform accordingly. According to Drill Sergeant Michael Johnson, "The tan boots are great for the soldier when we're deployed, but on the other hand those old black boots made inspections easy every morning. Highly shined boots didn't necessarily make a trainee a good private, but a good trainee would always have a good uniform. The boots were a good measuring guide. Now all trainees have to do is make sure they didn't step in the mud the day before, and they're home free." It's perhaps not the worst of things.

Matt Riker went through basic just after they started issuing suede boots, and so he didn't have to shine them. Instead, "We had to buff them with a brush and a suede stick. Buff and brush. Some things didn't change, though: If they got dirty we'd have to clean them with soap and water, and then brush them. *If* they got dirty? These are army boots being worn by trainees going through training, often in the mud—they are supposed to get dirty. It was a dilemma for the training: If they didn't get dirty, you weren't doing your job, but if they weren't clean, you also weren't doing your job."

The Home Ranger:
The Homesick Blues

T HERE IS AN OLD story about the trainee who desperately wanted to get out of the service. He would walk around all day picking up every piece of paper and wrapper on the ground. As he picked up each one he would look at it, shake his head, and say, "This isn't it. This isn't it." The medics tried everything to get him to stop this obsessive-compulsive behavior, but nothing worked. He continued to pick up every piece of paper he found. The medics finally accepted the fact that he was mentally disturbed and gave him an honorable discharge. When his Drill Sergeant handed his official discharge papers he looked at them, smiled, and said with great satisfaction, *"Here* it is."

Not every trainee adjusts well to basic. Sometimes, enlisting seemed like a good idea at the time, but the practical aspects of it don't become apparent until basic training. When Drill Instructors begin yelling about everything, and you are forced to eat, shower, and relieve yourself with forty other people, the concepts of service and sacrifice seem significantly less attractive. In almost every cycle there are recruits who decide they don't belong in the military and want to leave. Holly Kale (navy, Great Lakes, 2003) admits, "For the first two weeks I asked myself ten thousand times,

'What have I gotten myself into?' I cried every day for the first week. I had never experienced anything like this, but after a while I realized they weren't going to kill me, I was going to make it, and I began fitting right in."

Training Instructor Joe "Tuffy" Tofuri (air force, Lackland, 1961) will never forget one recruit who desperately wanted to get out of the service. "He had tried every excuse, but it was obvious he was faking. Finally, one night he confessed to my barracks chief that he was a werewolf and he was very concerned because there was a full moon that night. To prove his point he bit one of my trainees on the leg and started howling. When I heard about this I told the barracks chief to bring the kid to my office. When he reported he immediately dropped onto the floor and started howling, then growling at me. This was my first werewolf. And there is nothing in the TI handbook that tells you how to deal with a situation like this one. When I walked around my desk he suddenly pounced onto my leg and started gnawing on my combat boots. I didn't really know how to react, so I pushed him away. He apologized, explaining he couldn't help himself, that he was a werewolf. And this is what werewolves do."

Rising to the challenge, Tofuri asked him if he could change into any other animal. He said that he came from a long line of werewolves, his mother and father were werewolves, but that he could also turn into a bat. Oh, a bat, that was interesting. Tofuri knew he had him. "So let me ask you," he said. "Bats can fly; so can you fly?"

"That stumped him. When he admitted that he didn't know, I suggested an experiment. I opened the window in my office and grabbed him, one hand by his shirt collar, with my other hand I took his belt, and I started dragging him toward the window.

"That's when he stopped howling."

The behavior of recruits sometimes defies analysis. Kevin Kai

Johnson (navy, Orlando, 1976) had a boot who tried desperately to get out of the service. "This guy sneaked out of the barracks in the middle of the night, went over a barbed wire fence, and disappeared for a couple of weeks. It made no sense," he says. "At the time the navy policy was that if you didn't want to be there, all you had to do was tell them, and they would let you walk out of the gate."

The air force had a similar policy in the 1970s, remembers Olaf Casperson. "Until a certain point in training, you could just walk away. It was a free zone. But after that point you had to keep going. If you didn't keep up they recycled you into a new unit, and you had to start all over again. We had some people who knew they'd made a mistake. They couldn't adjust. They would cry themselves to sleep at night. Then all of a sudden there would be an empty bed and you'd never see these people again. No explanation, just gone. We started with about fifty guys and lost about ten of them during the cycle."

Without doubt, Michael Shapiro, at Ft. Dix in 1959, witnessed one of the most unusual unofficial absences reported anywhere. "One day about our third week this guy says to me, 'Listen, you got to do me a favor.'

"'All right,' I said. 'What is it?'

"'Well, I'm not going to be here for a few days and I need a little help.'

"Not going to be here? Okay. 'Going on vacation, are you?'

"He shrugged. 'You don't understand. Deer hunting season is opening in Pennsylvania and I don't want to miss it. But it's okay. My kid brother's going to take my place.' This was the strangest thing I'd ever heard, he needed a few days off from basic training so his brother was going to take his place. He explained, 'He's gonna drive my car onto the base. I'm gonna take the car and go deer hunting, and he's gonna stay with you guys.'

"Somehow, it actually made sense. And that's what happened: His kid brother drove onto the base, put on his clothes, and stayed about four days. We pointed him in the right direction and covered for him, and he got away with it until his brother came back. He actually took a vacation from basic training."

One recruit did successfully get discharged from Joe Lisi's Marine platoon at the height of the Vietnam draft in 1969, an extremely difficult thing to accomplish. "He just couldn't take it, and so he started wetting his bed. He'd heard that if you wet your bed they let you out. So he started wetting his bed. To prevent that, our DI ordered whoever was on barracks fire guard to wake him every two hours through the night. When that didn't work, they began waking him every hour. And when that didn't work, they began waking him up every fifteen minutes. But somehow he still managed to wet his bunk, and eventually they had to discharge him."

In the 1970s, there began a large increase in the number of women in the armed forces, and this presented problems not easily solved. Cindy McNally points out that women had a unique way of getting out of the air force in 1976. "Basic training was hard on a lot of women. For most of us, there was no way of preparing for it. But there was a regulation that if you got pregnant you were not permitted to stay in the military. The minute you got pregnant, married or single, you got kicked out. While the object of that regulation was to prevent women in the air force from getting pregnant, in fact it served the opposite purpose. Sometimes during what was referred to as casual time, free time, or when they were on leave, they would try desperately to get pregnant. I don't think they understood the equation: a few weeks of basic training versus a lifetime of raising a child."

When Bobby Oxford was at Great Lakes, he had a boot in his

platoon who desperately wanted to get out, so "He decided to play a trick. Just before an inspection he put a clump of peanut butter on the toilet seat. When the chief saw that, he demanded, 'What the hell is that?'

This kid stuck his finger in it, stuck it in his mouth and said, 'Shit, Sir.' We didn't see him after that, although I never found out what happened to him."

Before the military adopted its Don't Ask, Don't Tell policy, which allowed gays to serve as long as no one knew they were gay, there was a polite fiction that there were no homosexuals in the armed forces. Brian Dennehy remembers getting a lecture about it from the chaplain. "He said, 'There are some individuals who have this problem and they cannot be in the Marine Corps, but if you identify yourselves we will move you right out of training. We'll give you a discharge and you'll be sent home with an honorable discharge under medical conditions. It won't be a big deal.' We had one guy who just could not get with the program. He was always in trouble, always screwing things up. He wanted to get out and he decided that this was how he could get his honorable discharge. I remember him saying to us secretly, 'Watch, I'm getting out of here.'

"What he did was go in to see our DI and told him, 'I want to see the chaplain because I am a homosexual.'

" 'Really?' the DI asked.

"He was adamant about it. 'Absolutely.'

" 'All right,' the DI said, as he unzipped his fly and pulled it out. 'Prove it.' That poor guy didn't know what to do. He bolted out of that room and finished his training. We never had another problem with him."

Once it was quite common to have a few recruits go AWOL—Absent Without Official Leave—during the cycle. One day, often without any obvious reason, a recruit would just disappear. Drill Sergeant Shawn Herbella had "one female recruit who did everything correctly, passed every test, and never showed any signs of stress or not being able to get through. Then one night she decided to leave. She called her husband and had him pick her up on the side of the street and just left. There was no reason for it I could understand."

The Marines have a very effective means of preventing trainees from going AWOL on Parris Island—Parris Island. "The first thing they tell you when you get there is that there are only two ways off the island," remembers David Gregory Smith (Marines, Parris Island, 1996). "Through the front gate or through the swamps. And then they told you about the alligators in the swamps. You're on a marshy, mysterious South Carolina island and we believed everything they told us. When we were working out in the sand pits we could see the water and it was pretty obvious we weren't leaving until we dropped out or graduated."

A primary objective of basic training is to demonstrate to recruits that they are capable of withstanding far greater pressure than they imagined possible, a lesson that often proves invaluable later in life. Succeeding at something more challenging than anything you've ever countered can help build a strong foundation. No one really knows how much is too much until that point is reached. Failing to complete basic training can also change a life forever—and often in a negative way.

Of course, there were people who were equally dedicated, even desperate, to finish their training, among them Dennis Stead (Marines, Parris Island, 1960). To Stead, like so many others, basic training was a personal test, and the results of this test would influence the rest of their lives. "I desperately wanted to be a Marine, but I was way overweight. I was about 6'1" and before I went into the corps I was pushing 285. The Marine recruiter had an office in the Post Office and every so often I would drop in and tell him I was getting ready to join, on the assumption that if I made friends with him he would help me figure out how to get around the fact that I was overweight. He told me, 'Dennis, you got to get some of that weight off or we can't take you.' Losing weight became my focus. I went at it and lost about twenty pounds. Then the local pharmacist gave me some water pills that took about five or ten pounds of water weight off. I did whatever I could. Finally, I taped lifts on my heels underneath my socks. That gave me an extra half inch, which put me at 6'2" and let me carry another ten or fifteen pounds. I made it, I did it."

It's not enough to seem physically qualified. Marine boot camp is supposed to be very tough, and for Stead, being so big made it even more difficult. The intensity of the physical training made his weight a big liability, and eventually he was sent to the hospital. "My right knee started hurting badly, and I told the doctor that it hurt like hell. 'Okay,' he said, picking up that little metal hammer, 'Does it hurt when I tap it like this?' I came flying out of the chair. 'Okay, I guess it does,' he decided.

"They discovered that I had broken my kneecap. Several years earlier I'd been in a car accident, and I'd been thrown into the dashboard. It must have happened then and it hadn't healed correctly. They told me, 'We're going to recommend that you be surveyed.' I didn't even know what that meant, and they told me that I would be given a medical discharge under honorable conditions. 'The problem with an injury like this is that the bone chips could float. In combat it could possibly flare up, you wouldn't be able to move and you could get somebody else killed because of it.'

"I listened, but meanwhile I was thinking, 'No. No way. They can't do this to me. I spent too many years lugging my fat ass up the street to talk to the recruiters. I pleaded with the doctors, 'I've had a tough life here, guys, and I've gotta do this. You've got to let me stay.' I pleaded with them. 'I can't go home. I live in a small town, and if I don't complete this I'll be ridiculed. It'll turn my life upside down.'

"They listened, and I finally convinced them. The doctor told me 'I'm going to do something I'm probably not supposed to do. I'm not going to recommend you for a discharge. Instead I'm going to make a notation that you've got a bum knee that has to be watched. Within the next four years it's probably going to cause you too much pain or trouble and you'll get discharged, but at this point you're free to stay and be miserable.' I was in the hospital, I was in serious pain, but if there was one time I smiled, that was the day. That was the best news I'd heard. They were going to allow me to continue being miserable!"

Social Studies: Learning to Get Along

DRILL SERGEANT: Gump! What's your sole purpose in this army?

FORREST GUMP: To do whatever you tell me, Drill Sergeant!

DRILL SERGEANT: God damn it, Gump! You're a god damn genius. This is the most outstanding answer I have ever heard. You must have a goddam I.Q. of 160. You are goddam gifted, Private Gump. Listen up, people . . .

FORREST GUMP: (narrates) Now for some reason I fit the army like one of the round pegs. It's not really hard. You just make your bed real neat and remember to stand up straight and always answer every question with "Yes, Drill Sergeant."

DRILL SERGEANT: . . . Is that clear?

FORREST GUMP: Yes, Drill Sergeant.

—from the movie *Forrest Gump*, Paramount Pictures, 1994

I T IS A SAD and often frustrating truth that you don't get to choose your relatives, and in the military you don't get to choose your comrades. If you are purposeful, and creative with excuses, you can escape most relatives, but in basic training, you get no choice at all about the people you will work—or fight—beside. In the military you're stuck with your bunkmates, shipmates, and bunker-buddies, and in basic you have to learn to get along with everybody.

Drill Sergeant Ben Currin notes that, while there was at least one clown in every unit, he is one of the few instructors who actually had to train a clown. "I had a kid from Mt. Olive, North Carolina. Although I didn't know it right at the beginning, his daddy ran a hardware store and worked as a clown on the side, so naturally some of that rubbed off on his son. During serious moments he would be acting up, and so one afternoon I got up to him and demanded, 'Just what do you think you are, some kind of clown?'

" 'Yes, Sir!' he said firmly.

"I didn't realize he was being honest with me. Before enlisting he actually had earned money each weekend working as a clown at parties, but I didn't know that. I just thought he was being a wise guy. So I told him that we didn't have any clowns in the army, which as I soon found out wasn't completely accurate."

Rather than a clown, Richard Goldman went through Ft. Jackson with an actual genius. "He was some sort of mathematic genius who worked at NASA. He had a photographic memory, and he had read through the Army Manual and memorized all the rules and regulations. He was a tiny guy, maybe 5'5" and 100 pounds wet, but he knew all the rules. Maybe more importantly he also knew that our Drill Sergeants did not know the specific rules, and that gave him real power."

The behavior of Goldman's colleague was an early demonstration of how, in the military, audacity has real strength, and that in circumstances where all else may fail, size doesn't matter. Goldman said, "Apparently there was a regulation that mandated that trainees get a ten-minute break every hour. It was really funny watching him go right up to our 6'8", 300-pound Drill Sergeant, look him right in the chest, and tell him confidently, 'Drill Sergeant, we've been walking fifty minutes; the rules are quite clear about the fact that every fifty minutes you need to take a ten-minute break. I think we need to take a break.'

"And we would get a break. It was incredible. He made up the rules as we went along. I don't think any of our Drill Sergeants knew if the rules he quoted were real or if he was making them up, but they listened to him, and we loved him for that."

The military had its unique way of forging relationships, and the illogic of it could be stupefying. "Our Drill Instructors were constantly reminding us that we were Marines, that we never left anyone behind," says James Lambert (Marines, Parris Island, 1969). "We were responsible for each other. The entire system was set up to reinforce that concept. When one person made a mistake, we all paid for it." So far, so good. The notion that success in battle will be the result of community effort is easy to grasp and demonstrably true.

"But then," Lambert said, "the whole platoon would go out running and inevitably somebody would fall behind. If you stopped to help them the DIs would be all over you, screaming 'If he can't keep up that's his problem. Don't you go back and pick him up!' It was impossible to be right. We couldn't leave him, and we couldn't stop to help him."

For a lot of people, the strongest memories they will take away from basic training will be the relationships that they made, but in some instances those aren't particularly good memories. As Val Nicholas learned, the stress of basic changes people and sometimes causes them to make decisions they eventually regret. "I got stuck with a big fat guy who couldn't do anything. The one thing that was emphasized from the first day was that nobody gets left behind, nobody. So as his platoon leader, when he messed up, I had to do his push-ups. When he couldn't run, I had to drag him along. When he couldn't march, I had to carry his weapon. When the barracks had to be cleaned I'd assign him the simplest task: 'Just make sure there are no cigarette butts in the corner.' But when we were inspected they would find cigarette butts in the corner. Once we were at the firing range and he lost the firing pin to his M-16 in the sand, and so our sergeant made me go through that sand until I found his firing pin."

Leadership is complicated at the best of times, but in the military environment it can be inscrutable. It is especially infuriating because ultimately the mission is so very important to so many others. "In our sixth week the sergeant looked at him and said, 'You know, Nicholas has been riding you the whole time, don't you just want to slap him? Well, this is your chance.' And C—— gave me a very light slap to my chin.

"Then the sergeant said to me, 'Nicholas, C—— has been a pain in your butt this whole time. You go ahead and slap him.' I will regret what happened then forever. I hit that boy so hard he went flying, and for an instant I felt good about it. He just looked at me with complete bewilderment. I'll never forget that look on his face. Then the reality kicked in. I felt horrible. It wasn't his fault. He is who he is. As a leader it was my duty to figure out a way to make him better, not just punish him. It was a lesson I have never forgotten. Later I managed four departments at NBC Entertainment, and I never left a single person behind. No matter how poorly an employee performed, I found a place for them to excel. For me, the pain of hitting him never went away."

"Whenever you need me just ask for your buddy Jackie. And wherever I am, I'll get you. And if we have to cry together, we'll cry together. If we have to do push-ups together, we'll do 'em together. Okay? You remember that. You have to cry, you come get me so I can cry with you. Because we're gonna get through this together. I swear to God, we're going to get through this together. I can't make it through without anybody, you're not gonna make it through without anybody. We're gonna make it. We came in here to make it. We're gonna do it, we really are. Be strong, be strong. We're gonna do it, just remember that, we're gonna do it. Just keep it in your mind, we're gonna do it. Say it, say it. Keep on saying it, strong. We're gonna do it, we're gonna do it. We're gonna show these sergeants. And when graduation comes we're gonna throw our hats up so high and we're gonna be so happy and we're gonna go back to our block and everybody's gonna say, wow man, you really did it, you really did it. I didn't believe you had the guts to do it. And you're gonna be so proud, and when we come outta here we're not gonna be on the floor anymore, we're gonna stand tall and show people who we really are. When we come outta this place we're gonna be different. If we can get through this, we can get through anything."

—from the documentary *Soldier Girls*, by Nicholas Bloomfield and Joan Churchill

Except for the Drill Instructor, the one person a trainee gets to know better than any other is his "battle buddy." While the navy refers to this team as "shipmates," and the air force calls them "wingmen," the purpose is the same: Two or more people are a functioning entity, with each one of them responsible for the other. In most situations, the margin of victory is not the heroics of a single individual, no matter how laudable that might be, but instead the efforts of the group. According to *The Soldier's Blue Book*, "Soldiers rely on one another to stay motivated and reach peak performance . . . In

Initial Military Training, soldiers will form natural bonds with their fellow soldiers as part of the army culture. To contribute to this team spirit, we live by the buddy system . . .

"With the requirement to excel in army training, some soldiers need more positive reinforcement than others. For that reason you may also be paired based on your strengths, so you and your buddy can complement each other's weaknesses."

"On the first morning they marched us out into two rows and made us stand back-to-back," recalls Anthony Shaffer (army, Ft. Gordon, 1981). "They told us whoever we turned around to face was our battle buddy, and whatever happened we had to stick with him. I turned around and there was this black guy from Macon, Georgia, named Howard. We were worlds apart, we had absolutely nothing in common except we were facing the same challenges—but eventually we became really good friends."

Generally the system worked as intended. Nadine Gabrielle-Miran's (army, Ft. Leonard Wood, 1996) battle buddy was "A hot mess, an absolute walking disaster. She never made her bunk right, she always forgot to lock her locker, her uniform was always a mess, she was never squared away. Her idea of cleaning up was to shove everything into her locker and close the door. She came from a home where her mother took care of everything. I was responsible for her; I used to wonder why God was tormenting me.

"She would leave her locker open when the first sergeant came in to check the barracks. When he found an open locker he would take everything in it and throw it onto your bed, then throw all of your tampons around the room, and just to make sure everybody got involved, he would pull apart every bed in the room. There were six of us in that room, and when we came back at the end of our training day that place would be a total disaster."

It usually does not take very long before the group whose efforts are regularly destroyed by the incompetence of a single person decides to punish or eliminate the cause of the pain. In battle, with life and death on the line, sometimes that is necessary. In training it can be the basis of an important lesson. "Some of the people wanted to give her a blanket party, a beat-down," said Gabrielle-Miran, "but I told them we had to be compassionate. It turned out she had a lot of negative stuff going on at home. Instead, we worked together to get her in shape. We reminded her to check her locker, we made sure her bed was made properly, we cared about her problems, and eventually we brought her around."

Gabrielle-Miran had her own difficulties to deal with. "The toughest part of basic for me was shooting and throwing the grenade. My goal in joining the military was to go into the medical field, and so having a weapon in my hand for the first time and going out onto the range at below zero temperatures in February was a struggle for me. To pass, you had to be able to throw a grenade over a wall a certain distance, and I couldn't do it. First they gave you a ball the same weight as a grenade, and you kept throwing it and throwing it until you were able to get it over the wall. Then they tested you with a real grenade.

"I just couldn't do it. I threw it and ran. In fact, I'd be running before I threw it. Why wouldn't I? It was a grenade. It blew up. I was so nervous that I thought that as soon as the pin was pulled it was going to blow my hand off. I just threw it and ran.

"I was fortunate to have a Drill Sergeant who had patience. He worked with me for the entire week before graduation, teaching me how to focus, teaching me the proper stance. I just couldn't get it right, but he stayed out there with me in that bitter cold, and my battle buddies were right there encouraging me. 'You can do it, Gabby! You can do it!' I didn't want to go back out there in that cold, but they gave me their gloves, their extra scarves, whatever I needed. When I'd walk back inside they were right there, 'You get it this time?' Nope. 'That's okay, you'll get it next time.' It took me at least five times out on the course before I finally passed.

"At graduation we were all together, the girl that I had helped and all the girls who had helped me. We had built a very strong sense of camaraderie. We had been through it all together, and we all made it together. I can't really express how proud we were of each other."

That is, of course, the good news. But one of the most enlightening things about basic is that it exposes the average person to an extraordinary range of personalities. This is an education that can't be duplicated in any other environment, but on occasion it gets pretty frustrating. Michael Johnson believes that he may have had the worst possible battle buddy in basic training history. "There were twin brothers who bunked right next to me, and I got stuck with one of them. Both of these guys were just horrible. It would be hard to convey accurately just how awful my battle buddy was. I tried to help him make his bed, and keep his equipment in order, but neither of the brothers cared the slightest bit about getting it right. In fact, I'd be showing my battle buddy something, trying to get through to him, and while I was talking to him his brother would come up behind him and start popping pimples on his back. And that was the best thing about the two of them.

"These brothers were always doing something wrong and the whole platoon paid for it," Johnson reported. "As a penalty our DIs would make us do things like holding a full canteen out in front of us with our fingers through the loopholes. And just hold it there. And hold it there. If we lowered our arms they jumped all over us. You have no idea how heavy a full canteen can be after only a minute or two. People really struggled to hold it up; when you looked around the barracks everybody's face was turning bright red, you could hear people grunting, after a few seconds their arms would start shaking, but everybody gave a total effort.

"Everybody, of course, but these two brothers. After holding them up for a few seconds they just very nicely placed their canteens down on the floor. It was unbelievable. They just put them down as if doing nothing wrong. Naturally our sergeants then would take it out on everybody else. Finally I couldn't take this guy anymore. The sergeants knew what was going on and eventually they let me pick a different battle buddy."

The Real Battling Buddies:
Not Everybody Gets Along

Putting a large group of young people together in a stressful situation for a prolonged period is going to result in some conflict. Tempers are stretched taut during training, and it doesn't take much to ignite a fight or an argument. This is often the case when, as a way of teaching group responsibility, the entire platoon can be penalized for the actions of one individual—which is exactly what happens in combat. So things that normally would be trivial become incredibly important. Mike Volkin (army, Ft. Leonard Wood, 2001) was awakened one night by a brutal fight in the hallway. "Five weeks into the cycle these two guys went at it because one of them had been caught stealing the other one's underwear. I went out in the hall and there was blood all over the walls. The fight only lasted a few seconds but it resulted in two broken noses and a finger that was almost severed. Both of them were recycled and had to start at the beginning. It was obvious they hadn't learned all the lessons."

It isn't just male recruits who battled, either, at least according to Tracy Harwell (air force, Lackland, 2000). "Sixty women in one barracks was not a good idea. They just could not get along, and there was a lot of fighting. I was the dorm chief so I never got a minute's peace. It seemed like every time I turned around I was being called to break up a fight or settle an argument. I can't stand a lot of bickering, so it really pushed my patience.

"Some of the fighting was over amazingly petty things. For example, there was a thin chrome strip on the floor of our doorway, and it had to be shiny all the time. If it wasn't, we got some sort of extra duty, and so keeping that chrome strip shiny became extremely important to all of us. We got used to yelling to people when they came into the barracks, 'Step over the chrome!' Well, one day a girl accidently stepped on the chrome. She stepped on the chrome!

"The girl in charge of keeping the chrome clean completely freaked out. It was as if a terrible crime had been committed. She stepped on the chrome strip! It became a major fight that I had to break up."

Some of these fights can lead to serious consequences. Ken Dusick (army, Ft. Ord, 1969) woke in the middle of the night just as one recruit was holding a bayonet to the throat of another recruit. "Three of us grabbed him, disarmed him, and dragged him to the captain's office. The captain was a square-jawed Vietnam veteran. We described what happened and he said, 'Well, what are you bringing him to me for?'

"I said that it just seemed like the right thing to do.

"He then explained the facts of military life to me. 'If I have to report it to my commanding officer it looks like I have a company that I can't control. That's not a good thing for me. And if it's not a good thing for me, then it can't be a good thing for you.' When I asked him what we should do, he said, 'If it was up to me I'd just take him back inside and beat the holy crap out of this slimebucket.'

"Which is exactly what we did."

A Clean Start: Personal Hygiene

O F ALL THE CAPABILITIES of animals, the sense of smell, particularly in mammals, is the most highly developed—except
among human beings. Humans average about five million scent re-
ceptors, but dogs, for example, have more than two hundred million.
Although we can't detect odors very well, there is a limit to this in-
sensitivity, and stuffing large numbers of young people—some of
whom have had only a passing experience with a bar of soap—into a
relatively small area will quickly exceed even our low threshold.
During World War II, my father, David Jacobs, was training at Camp
Crowder, Missouri, miles away physically—and culturally—from his
home in Brooklyn, New York. Some of the trainees were from the
local area, which was in the Ozarks. "They were illiterate, and, so to
make sure these guys could read the Articles of War, they had to be
taught how to read and write," my father said. "But the biggest problem was that some of them never showered, and they created a really
unpleasant aroma in the barracks. Eventually they would get thrown
in the shower with all their clothes on. They figured it out pretty
quick."

Irwin Hunter had a somewhat similar experience in 1944 at New
York's Camp Sampson. "There was one guy from Maine who was

the single dirtiest man I had ever met. He never took a shower. I mean, never. He didn't even have to walk into a room for us to know that he was there. One day we decided to give him a little scrub down. We dragged him out of bed into the shower and rubbed him down with soap. He didn't like it too much, but we really didn't have much choice."

It wasn't just men and it wasn't only decades ago that trainees had to deal with this problem. "We had one girl who had no interest in personal hygiene," says Melissa Johnson (army, Ft. Sill/Ft. Leonard Wood, 2002). "Not only didn't she like to shower, she wouldn't wash her uniforms. You could see salt stains from her rucksack. She was really dirty. Finally we had to give her a GI Party. We dragged her into the shower, covered her with body soap, conditioner, shampoo, and rinsed her off. We gave her a good bath. And then we told her we would do it again if she didn't start keeping herself clean. After that she wasn't perfect, but she was better."

Hors D'oeuvres Are Not Served at Blanket Parties

A BLANKET PARTY IS a platoon's way of saying to an individual, stop screwing up. There are no invitations and, certainly, RSVPs are not required. A blanket party can be a pretty brutal means of sending a message, but it is almost always effective. The exercise goes something like this: In the night a group of people throw a blanket over the offending trainee, so he can't struggle and so the perpetrators can't be identified, and then beat him, painfully and convincingly, but usually never badly enough to send him to the hospital. This fine line is difficult to discern, and so a blanket party requires some skill, and even art. They are officially prohibited, and truthfully they rarely take place any more, but countless recruits have attended one or more of them. "A blanket party was kind of like the boogey-man," explains Matt Farwell (army, Ft. Benning, 2005). "It was meant to scare those people who were causing problems for the rest of the platoon, 'You'd better be careful or we're going to throw a blanket party for you, and you won't like it.' But it definitely was more of a means of scaring people than a real threat."

"Blanket parties were a tradition at Parris Island. They were commonplace," Thomas Kilbride remembers. "Like hazing in college. It's not something that goes on too much today, but it did, and it probably made people stronger. It was a pretty strong way of making the point that this recruit better shape up. I participated in a few myself. I'm not proud of it today, but when you're very young, it's almost a joke. The person who got hit one night might participate in giving somebody else a blanket party another night."

The army held them, too. Paul Steingruby III remembers, "A lot of times platoon justice would be meted out in the middle of the night. I never participated in one of them, but there were times I'd keep my head down, and I could see somebody who really got the whole company in trouble get ganged up on. He would be hit with fists or boots or whatever. But it was effective. The next day they would shape up."

His father, Paul Steingruby Jr. (army, Camp Carson, Colorado, 1957) had a similar experience. As might be expected when a large group of people is randomly thrown together, there are going to be conflicts. There are going to be people who don't get along, and sometimes that can prove dangerous. As Steingruby Jr. emphasizes, "There are always some people who plain don't like each other. I had a background in amateur wrestling, and so I got picked to be one of the training platoon sergeants, which meant I had a responsibility to maintain some type of order. The night before graduation a group of people decided it was their last chance to get even with another trainee. I don't know what their argument was. I just remember they had a blanket over this guy and they were beating him and kicking him. I went down there with another trainee sergeant and we were pretty powerful. When they saw us coming they scattered. After that I went to the orderly room and reported the incident.

"The next thing I know I was being told that two of the people involved in the beating were saying that they were going to kill me and the other person who broke it up as soon as we went to sleep.

I did consider it a real threat, I knew that at least one of these guys had enlisted instead of going to jail. I didn't feel like I could ignore that threat. So I went over and reported that, too. The Military Police came into our barracks and pulled those two people making the threats. They were held back from graduation and did not get to go home the next day, although I never found out what happened to them."

Kevin Johnson (navy, Orlando, 1976) also stopped a blanket party one night. "There was a small group who didn't like the way some of our platoon leaders were exercising control. So they decided they were going to hold a blanket party. Some of us got wind of it and made a point of informing them as nicely as possible that our platoon leaders were doing a very good job of leading—and the real problem was that they were doing a poor job of following. And after informing them nicely we added what was going to happen to them if they proceeded. That ended their plans right there, and after that night everything got settled down."

The Marine Corps Hymn

G OOD NIGHT, CHESTY PULLER, wherever you are!"
This is a common refrain said by Marine trainees when they hit the rack at night. Lieutenant General Lewis "Chesty" Puller was among the most decorated Marines in history, having been awarded five Navy Crosses. He enlisted during WWI, trained at Parris Island, and saw combat in Haiti, Nicaragua, in several of the bloodiest battles of World War II, and Korea.

"I Need Three Volunteers,
You, You, and You."

The foundation of military service revolves around the notion of being a volunteer. It was at the heart of our revolution, and even during periods when the country relied on the draft, a large percentage of those in uniform were volunteers. Once in uniform, the single most valuable piece of advice anyone who has served in the military can give to people about to enter basic is "Do not volunteer, ever. Whatever you do, do not volunteer." According to legend a Drill Sergeant once asked his platoon, "Anybody here know shorthand?" Three recruits immediately raised their hands, assuming this might be a way of getting out of training. "Good," the Drill Sergeant said, then ordered, "Get over to the mess hall. They're short-handed."

Ralph Strauss (army, Ft. Knox, 1945) learned this lesson one Friday night when his Drill Sergeant said, " 'Hey, we need a couple of guys who know how to drive a car. Raise your hand if you have a driver's license.' Driving? We all thought this was a good way of getting out of the barracks. About a dozen of us raised our hands and the sergeant picked out five of them. Then he brought them outside where they spent the rest of the night driving wheelbarrows loaded with dirt and rocks."

Anthony Shaffer (army, Ft. Gordon, 1981) developed his own strategy for avoiding "volunteer" details, explaining, "People warned me never to stand in the front if I could avoid it because they were always going to look for volunteers. It turned out to be exactly the opposite. The Drill Sergeants knew people were hiding in the back so they always picked their volunteers from the rear. If you were right up there in front they always avoided you."

Among the wisest counsel about volunteering came from an unknown Marine trainee who advised, "Never, ever, under any circumstances, in any way, tell the platoon sergeant you have nothing to do."

A Site for Sore Bodies: A Brief History of Training Sites

"Wait, this is not my life—I'm supposed to be at the boot camp on the beach with the spa!"

—*Private Benjamin*

Fт. Benning, Georgia, is named after Confederate Army Brigadier General Henry L. Benning, who was known to his troops as "Old Rock." He was a strong supporter of slavery and distinguished himself in several Civil War battles. Ft. Benning was established in 1918 to train troops for World War I. It covers more than 183,000 acres and is the country's largest basic training facility.

Ft. Jackson, South Carolina, is named for President Andrew Jackson, who as a major general led troops to victory in the War of 1812's Battle of New Orleans. Founded in 1917, in addition to recruits, it also has served as a training base for carrier pigeons, war dogs, cavalrymen, balloon and aircraft pilots.

Founded in 1940, Ft. Leonard Wood, Missouri, is named for Major General Leonard Wood, who began service in the 1880s Indian Wars as a surgeon and eventually received the Congressional Medal of Honor for valor. During the Spanish-American War

General Wood later commanded the Rough Riders and after his promotion was succeeded by his second-in-command, Teddy Roosevelt.

Ft. Bragg, North Carolina, was named after the commander of the Confederate Army of Tenessee, General Braxton Bragg. It was established in 1918 as a field artillery training center. Like many military bases, the site was appealing mostly because it was in a desolate area and has gained renown as the home of the Airborne Rangers.

Ft. Knox, Kentucky, was established at Camp Henry Knox, named after General Henry Knox, America's first Secretary of War and the Continental Army's Chief of Artillery during the Revolution. In addition to housing America's gold reserves in the United States Bullion Depository, during World War II the original U.S. Constitution, Declaration of Independence, Bill of Rights, the British Crown Jewels, the Magna Carta, and the gold reserves of several European nations were stored there for safekeeping.

Ft. Sill, Oklahoma, was laid out in 1869 by General Philip Sheridan, who named it after his West Point classmate, Brigadier General Joshua Sill, who was killed in one of the bloodiest battles of the Civil War, the Battle of Stones River. Apache Chief Geronimo surrendered there and lived out his life farming and selling autographs. It also is a National Historic Landmark.

A dry dock, the commanding general's residence, and a gazebo at the Marine Corps Training Depot at Parris Island, South Carolina, are also on the National Register of Historic Places. Parris Island was named after Colonel Alexander Parris, the third known owner of the island after it was settled by the British. Marines were first stationed on Parris Island in 1891, which was known until World War I as Port Royal, when a security detachment consisting of one sergeant, two corporals, and ten privates arrived there and soon attracted attention by saving lives and property during hurricanes and tidal waves that hit the island, but it was designated the East Coast Training Depot in 1915. The entire island was claimed by the government in 1918, when it was described by the Bureau of Yards and Docks—accurately, as anyone who has been there will agree—as 6,000 acres, "3,000 acres high and 3,000 acres marsh." Until 1929, when a bridge opened, it could be reached only by ferry. A separate command to train female recruits was activated in 1949. The most widely known feature of Parris Island is those marshes, or swamps. Dwayne Duckworth (Marines, San Diego, 1948) served as a Drill Instructor on Parris Island in the 1950s. "It was a hell hole. It was pretty primitive back then. We had a main base, but also had a lot of tents and huts. Everything was temporary. Except the swamps, the swamps were always there waiting, there was nothing like those swamps. I would take my troops down there on an afternoon but you'd have to be a little crazy to take them there at night. There were snakes and alligators in those swamps, in fact one of my recruits caught a king snake that must have been six feet long. It was harmless but there were other things in those swamps that weren't. Those swamps were bad all year round, but in the summer, you never forget being there."

Although Marines landed in San Diego in 1846 during the Mexican-American War and seized the town, the Marine Corps Recruit Depot San Diego wasn't commissioned until 1921. While East Coast Marine recruits stay at Parris Island for all their training, "Hollywood" Marines do their last weeks of field training at Camp Pendleton in San Diego County, the largest Marine base in the country, where they fire on the rifle range and go through the "Crucible," which tests their skills. Camp Pendleton was dedicated by President Franklin Roosevelt in 1942 and is named after Major General Joseph Pendleton, who was greatly responsible for the establishment of a West Coast Training Base.

President Theodore Roosevelt presided over the founding of the Naval Station Great Lakes, in Great Lakes, Illinois, which was officially opened in 1911. Prior to the integration of the military services, African American sailors were trained at Camp Robert Smalls, which was a section of Great Lakes named after a former slave who became a Civil War hero. Women didn't begin training at Great Lakes until 1994. Lt. John Phillip Sousa formed fourteen regimental bands at Great Lakes to entertain navy personnel. When the football team from Great Lakes beat Mare Island to win the 1919 Rose Bowl, the players—including future NFL founder and Hall of Famer George Halas, who scored both touchdowns and returned an interception 77 yards—were rewarded with discharges.

For seventy years, ending in 1993, the navy also trained sailors at the San Diego Navy Base, which also is listed on the National Register of Historic Places. An unusual feature of the 9-hole Sail Ho Golf Course on the base, which was once managed by recreation officer and golfing legend Sam Snead, is the graves of a former base commander and his wife—who might be said to have been buried at tee. The base also featured the USS *Recruit*, a two-thirds size model landlocked warship built in cement but actually commissioned in 1949. The USS *Neversail*, as recruits referred to it, was used to teach trainees shipboard procedures. As *The Anchor,* the base newspaper, described in 1971, "Although some seamanship skills only can be mastered from long experience at sea, the foundations upon which these skills are based form an important part of recruit training. Emphasis here is placed upon teaching recruits the language of the sea and the names and uses of the tools of his new trade. Among the subjects taught to the new recruit are marlinspike seamanship and knot tying, steering and sounding, anchoring and mooring, and the recognition of various types of ships, their characteristics, and structures. He learns the principles of shipboard organization and something of the role he will later play as a member of the ship's company . . .

"To facilitate practical demonstration of these subjects, the *Recruit*, a scale-model of a destroyer escort, was constructed on shore for use by the recruits. Onboard this landlocked ship practical exercises are held in stationing personnel in getting under way, in anchoring, for handling mooring lines, and the manning of watch and battle stations."

The base was officially closed in 1997.

Lackland Air Force Base, near San Antonio, Texas, was originally a section of Kelly Air Force Base known as "the hill," which was used for bombing practice. Construction began in 1941 but it wasn't until 1948 that it was named Lackland, after Brigadier General Frank Lackland, who was responsible for turning a former bombing range into the air force's only recruit training center.

The No Space Patrol:
Life in the Navy

IN ADDITION TO A uniform, during World War II a navy recruit was issued a hammock with a mattress, a mattress cover—which was also known as a "fart sack"—a pillow, cover, and two blankets. These items had to be stored in a sea bag, a canvas sack, with a line through the top so it could be hung from his rack. Aboard even the largest ships, space for personnel was at a great premium, and each sailor had less room for his personal use than that afforded to the average airline passenger traveling economy. Everything the sailor owned had to be stored in this sea bag, and the sailor essentially lived out of it.

As with all things military, trainees got no vote on procedure, and there was a prescribed way to pack it correctly. Clothing had to be rolled, tied, and put into the bag in a specific order, which helped reduce wrinkles and packing time, so that, when a sailor traveled, all he had to do was pick up his bag, sling it over his shoulder, and he was on his way. Irwin Hunter remembers, "All the clothing we were issued had holes in the waist band or legs, so after being washed, we could tie them to a clothing line to dry. We did have to scrub our own underwear and socks. I used to wear my shorts and T-shirt when I took a shower, then wring them out and hang them."

But the world, technology, and the services have changed. The need to roll clothes and live out of a sea bag ended in 1953, when boots in San Diego were issued lockers, and in any case many of the clothing items now issued to trainees by all services are made from wash and wear, permanent-press fabrics.

Myth #2: The Time-out Card

Drill Instructor Fitch: *(begins hitting recruit repeatedly on the head)* All right, cum-for-brains. Show me exactly where your skivvies and running shoes go.

Recruit: Sir. The recruit can't think when the Drill Instructor's hitting him on the head, sir.

Drill Instructor Fitch: You can't think when I'm giving you a few love taps? How the fuck are you going to fire your rifle when grenades are going off in your face? What the fuck are you even doing here?

Recruit: I got lost on the way to college, sir!

—from the movie *Jarhead*

THE TIME-OUT CARD: VIEWED from outside, much of basic training seems petty and counterproductive, serving primarily to denigrate and instill fear. Most people who have been through it will attest to its value—and later in life look back on it as an extraordinarily valuable experience. Unfortunately, there have been situations in which the tough love served in basic crossed the line and became dangerous maltreatment, and there have been instances in which recruits have been injured.

"The stuff that they did when I went through basic or when I was a TI that we got away with, they wouldn't even think about doing today," Mike Harrell (air force, Lackland, 1961) says. "Today there is too much attention on maltreatment. Some of the things we did that never hurt anybody would now be considered maltreatment and be prohibited. They even came up with a Time-out Card. If a TI got to chewing out a troop, and the troop thought it was going too far, all he had to do was flash this card. The TI had to stop. Believe me, there was no way in hell any one of my TIs would stop chewing me out because I flashed a card at him."

"They were called stress cards in the army," explains Shawn Herbella. "It's a plain card that you kept in your breast pocket, and if you got stressed out too much because the Drill Sergeants were yelling at you, or you got to the point where you couldn't handle it anymore, you would hold up this card and then they'd have to stop for five or ten minutes to calm down. I never saw one."

He never saw one because there was no such thing as a stress card in the army, even though the myth persists to this day that there was. Supposedly this card was yellow and for many people that color was symbolic of what it meant. The belief in the existence of a "stress card" was probably based on a blue card the navy issued to recruits during boot camp in the 1990s. Concerned that trainees were suffering from depression, which led to poor performance, going AWOL, or suicide attempts, the navy wanted boots to know that help was readily available. This "Blues Card" listed those places a recruit could go for help when things got too tough. It read: "In the Dumps? Thinking about giving up? Thinking about running away? Help is only a question away." After these cards had been in circulation for only a few months, navy instructors began reporting that recruits would wave them when being disciplined to signal they needed a time out. In response, the navy withdrew the cards.

At about the same time, the army issued cards to recruits, instructing them what to do if one of their buddies seemed greatly depressed, maybe even suicidal. ACE cards, as they were known, urged recruits to Ask your buddy, Care for your buddy, Escort your buddy. So while there never was a real stress card, the myth lives on.

Meet General Inspection:
It's Pretty Neat

"Why is there trash in my trash can?"
—a DI in the documentary *Soldier Girls*, Nick Bloomfield
and Joan Churchill

The oftener the soldiers are under the inspection of their officers the better; for which reason every morning at troop beating they must inspect the dress of their men; see that their clothes are whole and put on properly; their hands and faces washed clean; their hair combed; their accoutrements properly fixed, and every article about them in the greatest order. Those who are guilty of repeated neglects in these particulars are to be confined and punished.

Every Saturday morning the captains are to make a general inspection of their companies.
—Baron von Steuben's Revolutionary War Drill Manual

A T NO OTHER TIME in your life will you be more organized, cleaner, or more shipshape than during basic training. There is a proper place for everything, and everything, from the barracks floors to equipment, must be kept absolutely spotless. An essential aspect of teaching recruits to live in the military fashion is inspections, and consequently every aspect of a trainee's life is inspected—and re-inspected. Instructors use inspections as a teaching tool, basically to teach recruits that it's impossible to pass an inspection. "My biggest challenge in the navy was the superstrict bunk inspections and correctly folding my watch cap," according to Philip Landon (navy, Great Lakes, 2006). "The navy stressed attention to detail to the umpteenth degree. The amount of responsibility they gave you was extraordinary, and believe me the small things matter. So to reinforce that they focus on getting the small things right in boot camp."

"That attention to detail was really important," says Casey Gonzalez (navy, Great Lakes, 2007). "Your belt buckle had to align perfectly with the crease in your pants, for example. They even inspected the inside of your uniform sleeves and if you had a thread hanging that you hadn't burned off with a lighter, that was a serious problem."

Air force inspections were no easier, remembers Adam Mandlebaum (air force, Lackland, 1970). "They literally inspected the inside of our toothpaste tube and the inside of our shoeshine wax. We had to clean it with a Q-tip."

There is a tendency to deride such petty tactics as a misguided attempt to return to a different, tougher time, before we became enlightened. When Benjamin Franklin warned, "We must indeed hang together, or most assuredly we shall all hang separately," he certainly wasn't referring to uniforms hanging in a clothes locker, but his call for "uniformity" certainly is applicable. A lot of instructors use inspections to teach teamwork: In many situations, when one person fails an inspection the entire platoon is punished for it, and so everyone has to work together or suffer together.

"Our objective was to force recruits to figure out how to work together," explains Drill Sergeant Kevin Robert Meade. "We knew we could always find something, but what we looked for inside the barracks was a sense of uniformity. If your buddy is the same as yours, and you were the same as the guys across the room, you were good. That meant you were communicating throughout the entire platoon. We were trying to teach recruits that it isn't a two-man army, you need to go outside your comfort zone and work with everybody else or the entire army is going to fail. That's why I was much harder when it came to small things than I was about cleaning a weapon. I knew the weapon was going to be clean, but I needed to make sure each recruit understood that as a soldier they were part of a team and had to work as a team."

Air force Training Instructor Mike Harrell used that emphasis on group responsibility to bring his training platoon, his "flight," as it is known, together. "I had one kid straight off the Navajo reservation. At the beginning he was absolutely lost. Everyone would be mingling around the barracks, talking and working together, and this kid would be sitting on the end of his bunk by himself, his head down like he didn't want to be noticed, shining his boots or getting his locker squared away. He was always by himself, and I felt so sorry for him I could cry. I had a conversation with my dorm chief and I told him, 'You've got to do something so this kid starts to open up.' So he and a few others began going over to him and asking, 'Your locker really looks up tight, you mind helping me with mine?' By the end of training he was right there among them, talking and laughing. You can't imagine how good that made me feel."

In basic, everything counts and, as Olaf Casperson (air force, Lackland, 1978) learned there are penalties for failing an inspection. "Everything had to be perfect. TIs had to be able to bounce a quarter on your bunk, your locker had to be squared, and even if you got all that right, if they wanted to they would find a problem.

Near the end of basic training we were scheduled to have our first leave. We were planning to go into San Antonio, and I was really looking forward to it. For some reason they had a policy that you had to write down the serial numbers of every bill you were carrying on a piece of paper and carry it with you. Without thinking about it I'd spent a dollar to buy shoeshine polish. When we were inspected the TI discovered that I'd spent a dollar and hadn't crossed it off my list, and so while everybody else went into San Antonio, I spent the weekend sitting in the dorm. That's how tough they were."

It would not be accurate to say that a recruit's life and possessions are an open book—because even an open book would be enough to cause a trainee to fail inspection. Kihm Winship (air force, Lackland, 1968) reports that his recruiter gave him essential and accurate advice, "He told me that if I wanted to take any addresses or photos with me, to tuck them into a Bible, because that was the only thing they wouldn't confiscate. One of the first nights a TI we didn't know came through, assisted by two recruits carrying pillow cases. He went from man to man and searched each foot locker. He pulled out my copy of *The Hobbit* and asked what it was. Fantasy, I said. He threw it into the pillow case, 'Well, you won't be needing that here.' Then he picked up my copy of the Bible, in the back of which were all the addresses of my friends and a photo of my girlfriend. 'What's this?' he asked. 'That's the Bible,' I said. It was like magic. He looked at it for a moment longer, snorted with frustration, handed it back to me, and moved on to the next man."

Instructors would look for the smallest item out of place. "Folding every item perfectly and putting it exactly in the designated place in your sea locker was one way of teaching discipline," remembers Doug Kasunic (navy, San Diego, 1963). "There was a proper place for everything, whether it made sense or not. When we had locker inspection we'd be standing at attention, and the commander would walk by, and if he found one thing out of line in one foot locker, then he'd dump everything out of everybody's locker and tell us to redo it right. Everybody paid the price. There was always somebody out of line, and we'd end up refolding our dungarees, refolding our socks, refolding our hats."

As Paul Setmaer recalls, air force trainees had security drawers in their lockers. "When we got to Lackland they gave us a book that told us how to fold your towels correctly and hang your shirts and uniforms. Who knew there was an incorrect way to fold a towel? There was a security drawer in our locker, and we were supposed to put everything of value we had in it. Everything. There was a specific place in that drawer for your wallet, your spare change, stamps, anything of value. During our first inspection our TI found a letter one of the trainees had written to his girlfriend, but he'd made a bad mistake: He put a stamp on it. As the TI pointed out, loudly, the stamp had not been cancelled, and so it still had value, and since it had value it should have been in the security drawer.

"He proceeded to rip apart this airman's locker. Then the TI handed him the security drawer and for the rest of the inspection, at least an hour, he had him marching throughout the two bays screaming, 'Your valuables belong in your security drawer, your valuables belong in your security drawer.'"

Much like some people would sleep on top of their bunk once it had passed inspection, and then tighten it again in the morning, once a foot locker passed inspection some trainees would never touch it again. "People would live out of their laundry bag," explains David Taylor (air force, Lackland, 1968). "Once my foot locker finally passed inspection, it was never changed and remained in perfect order. I had a whole system. I kept my clean laundry stuffed into the bottom of a laundry bag. Our laundry bags had a drawstring closure at the top and a zipper at the bottom. I would put dirty laundry in the top, so that if our instructor looked in there he'd see the dirty stuff, and I would pull clean laundry out of the bottom. So I never had to learn all the tricky folding patterns or remember precise positions in my foot locker. One time we had an inspection the same day I did laundry, and so everything I had was clean; to avoid getting caught, I polished the floor with my clean laundry and then put it right on top of my laundry bag.

"My sergeant knew I had to be doing something because nothing ever changed in my foot locker, but he could never figure it out. He would spend more and more time each inspection checking my locker, but he never was able to catch me."

Taylor found a relatively simple but effective solution to the dilemma of having to live an active life while concurrently being inspected for adherence to an ideal of perfection. He was fortunate he didn't have Tim Price, who was at Lackland at the same time, as his TI. As Price says, "We knew we had guys living out of their laundry bag. They'd continually change between one pair of clean underwear and a pair of dirty ones. But eventually we figured out how to catch them: The clothes in the bag would accumulate dust on them."

John Langeler (navy, Great Lakes, 1966) found that group punishment for an individual's failure was a tremendous motivational tool. "One morning we had to get dressed in a big hurry. It seemed like we were always in a big hurry to get to a place so we could stand around and wait while nothing happened, but that morning we got dressed and raced to the drill field for an inspection. They came down the line and I was ready for them. I knew I was squared away. I was going to pass this inspection. Then the chief petty officer yanked down the front of my turtle neck and asked me why I'd put my T-shirt on backwards. Backwards? These things had no labels, we were racing to get dressed in the dark and it was under a turtle neck. I couldn't even figure out how he knew it was back-wards. When the inspection was done the chief announced that everyone would have to do an hour of close order drill because that 'fucking idiot Langeler put his T-shirt on backwards.' For the rest of the day everybody hated me. But believe me, I never put a T-shirt on backwards again."

At Ft. Sill in 1944 Jerry Leitner remembers instructors making certain that trainees put their underpants on the right way. "They used to tell us that it was easy to find the front and back of under-pants. The yellow stains went in the front and the brown stains were in the back."

TI Mike Harrell was once faced with his own underwear di-lemma. "I had a recruit come in, and that first night as they were get-ting undressed I noticed he was wearing the strangest underwear I have ever seen. They looked like a half-set of long johns, cut off midthigh. I asked him, 'Son, what are you wearing?' And he said, 'That's my underwear.' Then he explained that he was a Mormon, and in that religion married men had to wear this type of underwear.

"Okay, but that presented a problem for me. Each recruit had a wall locker and two drawers, and every single thing in there was supposed to be hung a certain way, folded a certain way, and placed in a certain spot to comport with regulations. I didn't know how I was going to work out this display with his special underwear. The thing we teach is uniformity, and this was very different.

"I went to my supervisor for an underwear conversation. Turned out he had heard of this problem before and said, 'Here's what you do. Have him take his regular issue clothing, fold it the way it is supposed to be folded, and put in the right place. Then keep the stuff he wears in his laundry bag. But keep the stuff in the drawers for inspection.'" In other words, as Harrell was told, bend the rules a little bit: Let him keep his drawers in his drawers.

Adherence to military regulations governing personal appearance is essential, and recruits are regularly inspected on all aspects of it. For some people, that has proved to be a problem. These regulations have almost no comparison in civilian life. Many young people enter basic training having led lives that, in terms of appearance, can most adequately be described as casual—especially concerning facial hair. Even if a recruit's whiskers are thin, slow-growing, and on occasion prepubescent, shaving is an important part of the trainee's daily routine and permits them to prove that they are red-blooded Americans, literally. There are few easier ways of failing an inspection than shaving improperly or not closely enough.

Kellee Ryan (air force, Lackland, 1988) recalls her TI "telling our mixed flight what he expected. As an example he told us about another flight of newbies who he ordered to get upstairs and shave off all the hair on your face. Apparently they took him literally. 'When they came back,' he told us, 'they were all completely clean-shaven, and all of them were missing their eyebrows.'"

Many trainees are too young to have shaved regularly, so the results of their initial efforts were predictably incomplete, inept, or bloody. "The first morning we were expected to get up, shower, and shave," explains Paul Setmaer. "I had nothing to shave. I just had a little bit of peach fuzz on my mustache area, but the TI expected you to perform a complete shave. At that time we didn't have safety razors. We had two-edged blades where you dropped the blade in and locked it in place. I slathered on lather and began shaving, I had typical adolescent acne and I cut myself in the strangest places. All of a sudden I saw blood popping up, and I thought I was cutting off my head. I thought in my attempt to appease this guy I was going to die.

"And then I had to worry about getting blood all over everything. The worries were endless."

Each morning the Drill Instructors would pick out those men

who had not stood close enough to their razors. On Parris Island in 1960, as Dennis Stead recalls, the Marine Corps had its own system for solving that problem. "The Drill Instructor said that it appeared we'd had a fight with Mr. Gillette—and lost—and therefore a punishment was in order. He had us get our razors and take the blades out, and then scrape it up and down the cement floor of our barracks. Then we put them [blades] back into the razors and gave ourselves what is called a 'dry shave,' meaning no soap, no shaving cream. And we did it the Marine way: We put on our helmets, stood on one foot and jumped up and down—and shaved. By the time we were finished we were gushing blood. It would a celebration for the Red Cross.

"Four or five of us paid the price, but the next morning the other eighty guys shaved like hell. There was never again the problem of not shaving well."

One morning Mike Volkin's (army, Ft. Leonard Wood, 2001) Drill Sergeant inspected him carefully then asked if he had shaved that morning. "I told him I'd shaved, but he accused me of lying to him. It was a freezing cold day, there was snow on the ground, but he ordered me to get down and start rolling in the snow. I had a real problem. 'Drill Sergeant,' I said, 'we just had a class in Army values and I'm not going to lie to you. One of those values is honesty and I swear I shaved this morning.'

"No matter how many times I told him I'd shaved he didn't believe me. I was stuck in a Catch-22. Should I lie to him after swearing I was telling the truth and agree that I hadn't shaved, or do I keep taking the punishment for being falsely accused? So I just kept doing push-ups until he got tired."

Mike Zaleuka wrote in his blog, "My Life in Army Basic Training," Ft. Benning, 2009:

"I don't know if you remember me telling you about my battle buddy a while ago when I first got here, but every day he seems to prove me wrong. When you think there is no possible way a person could get more stupid, it happens. The best way I could describe him would be Lloyd Christmas from *Dumb and Dumber*. Honestly, it's pretty damn close to that. He provides me with hours of endless laughter from day to day. Today while I was lying on my bunk writing a letter, he was passed out on the floor next to me. My friend Nick and I took a Sharpie and drew a sweet mustache and soul patch on him. About five minutes later we all had to head down to form up for chow, and after everyone laughed at him he realized there was something on his face. He saw it was a mustache and when we told him we had to go right now, he grabbed shaving cream and a razor to get off a Sharpie mustache. . . . That, ladies and gentlemen, will be the person who could be covering my ass in a firefight one day."

Michael Shapiro certainly witnessed one of the strangest inspections at Ft. Dix in 1959. "We had one guy in our platoon who may have been a genius—but he was completely untrainable. He could talk about scientific theories, but he couldn't figure out how to make up his bunk. It wasn't an act; he just couldn't figure out how to do the easy things. One morning we did the infiltration course. We were absolutely filthy, and we had an inspection scheduled for late that afternoon. At the noontime formation the captain called out this recruit and ordered him to return to the barracks and spend the afternoon preparing for the inspection. 'Before I leave the post today,' the captain said, 'I'm coming in to make sure you're prepared!'

"When we got back to the barracks this recruit was laying on his unmade bunk, reading. He hadn't done anything. So we all helped him get ready for it. Just as we finished, the captain walked in. Wherever the captain was going that night, he was dressed for it. He had on his class A uniform and looked very sharp. He inspected this recruit's bunk, his foot locker, his uniform. We'd done a good job, everything was squared away. We began thinking, holy cow, he's actually gonna pass this thing. The only thing left to inspect was his M-1 rifle. I was thinking, it's his rifle, what's the worst thing that can happen?

"The captain took the rifle from this recruit and, searching for lint and dust particles, closely inspected the front sight. "Good," he said. Then he peered intently down the barrel and pulled back the bolt—and with that about a gallon of oil came gushing out of the barrel all over the captain's spotless uniform.

"It was the funniest thing I had ever seen," says Shapiro, "but not one person made a sound. That room was filled with the loudest silence I have ever heard. But we were all thinking hysterically. The captain just stood there, oil dripping off his ruined uniform onto the floor, staring at this trainee. He didn't look angry, just astonished. The recruit stood there, staring straight ahead, as if nothing had gone wrong. The captain was so far beyond any rational response that all he could do was to hand back the rifle, spin on his heels, and walk out of our barracks. He never said a single word."

Probably the most widely known—and feared—type of military inspection is the legendary "short-arm inspection." Apparently this was never a regular feature of basic training, but everybody certainly knew about it. A short-arm inspection allowed medical personnel to check soldiers for sexually transmitted diseases. Every few weeks soldiers would be ordered out of their bunks in the middle of the night and stand for inspection dressed in boots, helmet liner, and an overcoat—and nothing else. Soldiers were ordered to stand at attention, in those circumstances an ironic choice of command. When ordered to "present" they ceremoniously but with great trepidation opened their coats and allowed the medical staff to inspect their "short arm" for any sign of STDs. Generally, because trainees might have been infected before entering the service, short-arm inspections were done early in basic training, but once there, troops almost never left the base, pretty much eliminating the need for this embarrassing procedure.

As a means of emphasizing teamwork, the entire platoon is responsible for not only themselves and their own equipment but the barracks as well. In Orlando in 1976, for example, Kevin Kai Johnston remembers that his squad would get an unsatisfactory rating if the chief petty officer—whose rank Johnston maintains was appropriate to the nit-picking he did during inspections—could slip a fingernail behind a tack on the cork bulletin board. "The things that suddenly matter to you are amazing. We had a group of five people who knew how to fold clothes and clean and organize and prepare the barracks for inspection. We were called 'the miracle squad.' Then we got hit with the round thumbtacks not being flush with the bulletin board. It mattered. So I would bang in each tack with my shoe to make sure it was level." As Johnston later added, eventually he would work as a nuclear reactor operator on a submarine, where paying attention to the smallest detail actually mattered. Maybe the chief petty officer wasn't so petty after all.

Steve Baudo was never certain if it was an advantage or disadvantage to share a two-man room at Lackland in 1964. "No matter how carefully the two of us cleaned that room, the TIs could find something wrong with it. I got in trouble several times for not having my socks rolled correctly or for imperfect folds in my bed. If they found anything wrong they'd pull the mattress off the bed and throw it on the floor, tear off the sheets, dump your drawer, and make you start all over again. And we'd get a punishment detail, an extra day of marching or KP or extra duty of some kind. But one day we knew we had it nailed, and that room was perfect. We were ready for anything they were going to look at. The bed was so sharp you could get a paper cut if you sat on it. I'd spent hours rolling every sock until it was perfect. I never thought I would take such pride in perfectly rolled socks, but I did. Then the inspector came in wearing white gloves—and the first thing he did was get up on his toes and rub his finger along the sill on the top of the door.

"Then he showed me his index finger, covered with dust. Who looks for dust on top of a door sill? He did, obviously. 'What's this?' he demanded. I wanted to scream at him, 'Look at my socks! You ever seen such perfectly rolled socks?' Instead, at that moment dust on the top of door sill had become the most important thing in my life. We'd failed. We hadn't dusted our door sill."

At Lackland, in preparation for inspection, airmen actually held "dust drills," in which one man shouts out commands that set everyone else to work: "Top of your wall locker! Windowsill! Side of your wall locker! End posts! Bed rails! Vertical rails! Horizontal rails! Between your bed and your neighbor's bed! Beneath your bed and your neighbor's bed," and as each command is shouted the squad attacks that place. It has been said that among the biggest mysteries of air force basic training is exactly where the dust bunnies of San Antonio are created, but one thing is for certain: Eventually they all migrate to your barracks.

At one time or another most trainees have fought a battle with the floor waxer—a battle many of them have lost. The floors of most barracks are so clean that you literally could eat off them, especially if you like the taste of wax. Mostly the floors are waxed and shined with an electric buffer, but to bring the barracks to inspection-grade sheen, trainees are often forced to use more labor-intensive methods. "When we first got to basic they gave us a can of neutral polish, a toothbrush, then we found some rags," Kevin Kai Johnston reports. "We got on our hands and knees and shined that floor one foot by one foot, square by square. We put on the wax with a toothbrush and buffed it up. By the time we were done that floor was beautiful."

Sammy Lee Davis vividly remembers the classic deep red linoleum floors at Ft. Jackson in 1966. "The first few days we went to the PX and bought a special wax and a baby blanket. We'd put on the wax and then buff it with that blanket. We weren't supposed to do it that way, and so we had to get up in the middle of the night to clean the floors. But as a result that floor was shining. In basic people take great pride in the floors. Of course, as we found out later our Drill Sergeants knew exactly what we were doing because we were doing the same thing every unit before us had done. The real secret in basic training is that there are no real secrets. One thing you eventually learn is that nothing happens in basic that the Drill Sergeants don't know about or want to happen."

Myth #3: Suicide by Buffer

A MONG THE STORIES TOLD most often about basic is the woeful tale of the despondent trainee who tried to commit suicide by floor buffer. A floor buffer is a large machine with a round, rapidly rotating brush pad that glides too easily over newly waxed floors. A buffer weighs about forty pounds, and most of them are equipped with a forty-foot-long power cord. Trainees have spent decades learning how to wrestle these high-speed, unbalanced machines. They are notoriously recalcitrant, with minds of their own. They are empowered with an otherworldly inertia, taking their own time to respond to pushing them in the desired direction, then forcing the operators to overcompensate. There are few natural masters of the buffer. According to this story, a despondent trainee lugged one up to the roof of his barracks and wrapped the cord around his neck. He then tossed it over the side of the building, expecting to be yanked over the edge. Instead, he heard the machine crash into ground with the long cord still sagging from his neck. According to this "absolutely true" myth, the trainee was forced to pay for the smashed machine—and from that night on, he had to wax the floors by hand.

But for most trainees that buffer is a lifesaver. Every night another coat of wax is put on the floor, often until the linoleum or, in some cases the cement, literally shines. Throughout the night there is always one barracks guard on fire duty, and part of that watch consists of buffing the floor. When the wax buildup is too much, then the wax removal detail goes to work. Some trainees have used the dull knives from their mess kits to strip the wax off the floor inch-by-inch-by-inch.

Maybe second only to the floors was getting the bathroom porcelain shining brightly. Trainees are well known for finding creative ways to make sinks and heads shine. Dennis Stead claims that when he was at Parris Island, trainees were not permitted to drink soda, "The only thing we were allowed to use it for was cleaning the bathroom. Turns out soda does a great job making porcelain shine."

This Man's Salami:
Contraband in the Barracks

"Send a salami to your boy in the army."
—Katz's Deli (New York) slogan

AMONG THE WORST POSSIBLE things that could happen to any trainee is to get caught with contraband in the barracks. Contraband, in this instance, is anything not specifically authorized by the regulations. James Chittenden (army, Ft. Sill, 1992) made the serious mistake of getting caught with an illegal substance. "I admit it. I had a one-pound bag of peanut M&Ms. When our commander found them I felt just like I had been caught committing a very serious crime. I couldn't believe it. About half the platoon was surprised that I could be so stupid as to get caught, but the other half thought I had unbelievable courage to try to smuggle M&Ms into the barracks! The commander held up the bag so that everyone could see it and asked me the question I didn't want to answer, 'What's this? What's this?'

"Never has the phrase 'M&Ms, Drill Sergeant,' sounded so frightening!"

One of the first warnings given to Andy McKee's platoon (army,

Ft. Leonard Wood, 2008) was not to get caught with contraband in the barracks. "They said, 'If you try to sneak it in here we will find it. We have been doing this for a long time, and we are way ahead of you.' We heard all the stories about the strange places that people had tried to hide things. Then another platoon found old cans of Pepsi and candy hidden in the ceiling. They knew this contraband had been there for a long time because the Pepsi logo had changed six or seven years earlier and this was the old logo. We didn't know whether to be more impressed by the fact that someone had successfully hidden stuff behind ceiling tiles for seven years or the fact that they'd found contraband hidden in the ceiling."

As every recruit eventually learns, contraband *often* is hidden in the ceiling, A fact that obviously is overlooked by instructors. A female going through boot camp in 1967 once reported finding a girdle hidden in the ceiling and claims she became very popular because, at six feet tall, she was the only trainee who could reach high enough to put things up there.

"Pogey" bait is the term used to describe any food, particularly candy, that has not been issued by the military. In training, pogey is all the good stuff you're not supposed to eat or drink. There are several explanations for the source of that phrase, but one is that Marines in China prior to World War II would use the candy issued in their K rations to trade with the Chinese. Loosely translated, the Chinese word for prostitute sounds like "pogey," and so candy became "pogey bait." Another explanation is that "pogue" is a term used to described someone working in an official capacity, usually some officious bureaucrat, and candy and sweets could be used to bribe him.

Whatever the derivation, pogey bait was not permitted in the barracks. As Steven Singer (army, Ft. Polk, 1970) learned, the last thing any recruit wanted to happen is to get caught with pogey bait.

"My older brother lived in Chicago, and he sent me a box from an upscale food place. I don't think he completely grasped the concept behind basic training: This box included salami, crackers, cheeses, and hard candy that he thought I would like to share with my friends while I was out of town.

"I don't think a salami ever created this kind of dilemma. On one hand I wanted to throw it out, but on the other hand it was a salami! So in what was clearly a moment of temporary insanity I hid this salami in my locker. About 4:00 A.M. one morning they woke us up for a surprise inspection. I stood in front of my bunk, and I felt like I was in a horror movie. I could see the Drill Sergeant coming closer and closer. He got to my locker and he found this pogey bait. Personally, I was always impressed by their creative use of the English language. The phrases they would use, the analogies, were really impressive. He started ranting and raving, and I thought it was phenomenal the way he would come up with new words.

"He finally took all my gourmet snacks and tossed them on the barracks floor for everyone to share before breakfast. As a result I ended up with three extra days of guard duty walking off my salami."

Ken Dusick (army, Ft. Ord, 1969) faced a similar dilemma, although in addition to a dried kosher salami he had hidden a *New York Times* in his locker. "One day our Drill Sergeant announced that ammunition was missing so they were holding a surprise inspection. They put us at parade rest and brought one trainee at a time into the barracks while his locker was searched. I stood there with the hair raised on the back of my neck: How many years was I going to do in Leavenworth for my salami?

"In other lockers they found ammunition, knives, even drugs— but then my turn came. The sergeant pulled out the *Times* and shook his head in disbelief. What kind of soldier reads the *New York Times*? Then he dug deeper into my locker and pulled out my mess kit and my beautiful, half-eaten salami. He looked at me and I said the first thing that came into my mind, 'There's a knife in my mess kit. Wanna try it?'

"He actually smiled. Then he cut off a piece, decided it was really good, and put it back in my locker."

Melissa Johnson's mother would send forbidden sweets to her at Ft. Leonard Wood in 2002. "One time the Drill Sergeant opened a package and discovered the candy. Uh oh, I figured, it's over for me. Instead he asked, 'Is this for me?'

" 'Well, it must be, Drill Sergeant,' I said, 'because it's definitely not for me!' "

Many recruits claim the most difficult part of the transition to the military was that smoking of any type was prohibited in basic training. "At the time I went to basic training I was a smoker," explains Shawn Herbella (army, Ft. Jackson, 2004). "I was forced to stop, but it was hard, really hard. I wasn't the only one and we were desperate for a cigarette. Sunday was picking-up-trash day. There were no real drills going on. So we would go around picking up discarded butts. There was a pack of matches in our MREs. We'd smuggle in those matches and collect the discarded butts and share them.

"I was addicted, and I would have done anything for a smoke. It was hard to get away with it because it stinks and it stays on your breath and they were always in your face. But finally I came up with a plan. Our family and friends were allowed to send us care packages, letters, whatever. I wrote to a friend and told him to buy some cans of shoe polish, empty them and put as much Copenhagen (chewing tobacco) in them as possible and seal them. That way the Drill Sergeants world think it's shoe polish. I thought it was a great plan.

"The Drill Sergeant opened all the mail to inspect it. When he opened my package four cans just went crashing down on the floor. Fortunately, none of them opened. But our DI was a little surprised. 'Hey Herbella,' he asked. 'How come your friend is sending you shoe polish when you can buy it right here? I mean, you can stock up on the stuff.'

Fully aware of the potential consequences, Herbella was shaking with fear. "'I don't know, Drill Sergeant,' I said. 'I guess he didn't know what to send.' The Drill Sergeant didn't open them. I had four cans of tobacco. I knew I couldn't smoke it, but at least I could get my nicotine fix.

"My close friends were ecstatic. I shared the first two cans. At night before lights out we'd shower and get ready for bed, and study our manuals. And then we'd sneak into the stalls and just sit there in bliss. After a few days I realized it was disappearing too quickly. If I was going to make it last I couldn't share it anymore. So I told my friends that I was sorry, but if this is going to last me till we're done I had to keep it for myself."

With Herbella laying claim to his own tobacco, his friends became desperate. "They started offering to pay me, as much as ten dollars for a single pinch. 'I can't,' I told them. 'I don't need the money, I just need to keep it for myself.'

"'Okay, twenty bucks.' I wasn't negotiating, I really wanted to keep it.

"'Forty bucks. Man, you're a tough negotiator.' I sold my first pinch for forty dollars. When word got around other people began coming to me. All I wanted to do was get myself a little tobacco, and the next thing I knew, with my shoe polish tins of chewing tobacco, I was running a major contraband operation. The price kept going up. In basic there was almost nothing on which the trainees could spend money, and so people had cash but nothing to buy." In a classic demonstration of both the law of supply and demand and the nature of addictive behavior, Herbella's fellow trainees began offering him large sums for a small taste of nicotine. "I had an offer for a hundred and fifty dollars a pinch. I didn't want to give it up, and I didn't want to be an asshole, but a hundred and fifty dollars? I probably made four hundred dollars on those last two cans of three-dollar dip. Most importantly, though, I never got caught with tobacco in the barracks."

Worse than getting caught with tobacco? Getting caught with ammunition. At Ft. Benning in 2004, Tom Burke explains, "We did a six-mile battle march-and-shoot. We had to run all that way with our flak jackets, at the end we had to fire our weapons. Until that time, throughout basic, they had always told us when to lock and when to reload, but this time they didn't do it. So one of our people didn't reload. Instead he put a fully loaded magazine in his flak jacket, brought it back to the barracks and stored it in his locker. When the Drill Sergeant found a magazine with thirty rounds in this recruit's locker, he explained honestly, 'Well, Drill Sergeant, I didn't know I had to shoot them.'"

Finally, David Taylor (air force, Lackland, 1968) remembers the oddest thing a Drill Sergeant ever found inside a foot locker was an actual, live recruit, who apparently had climbed in there to avoid the inspection.

The Drive for Success

FOR SOME REASON RICHARD Goldman (army, Ft. Jackson, 1968) never learned, his Drill Sergeant decided that he should have a military driver's license. "He said to me, 'In order to get your license you have to learn how to drive a jeep.' He decided he was going to teach me himself, and so we drove into the middle of woods. Then he said, 'Okay, you drive the jeep back to the barracks.' We were way out in the woods in Columbia, South Carolina, in the middle of the night, and it was pitch black. You couldn't see a thing, but if he wanted me to drive the jeep, I'd drive the jeep.

"I got behind the wheel and the first thing I did was turn on the lights. He looked at me like I was crazy. 'What are you doing?' he asked.

"It seemed pretty obvious to me, but if he needed an explanation I'd give him one. 'I'm putting on the lights so I can drive back to the barracks.'

"He reached over and shut them off. 'You can't do that. You have to drive without lights.'

It seemed obvious to Goldman that since it was dark and the vehicle had headlights, he should use them. Goldman didn't argue, figuring there had to be some military reason for not turning on the lights when you were driving in the woods in the dark. "I put the jeep in gear and took off. I got maybe eight feet and I crashed right into a tree. That actually wasn't much of a surprise to me. I was driving in the dark! The Drill Sergeant started screaming at me, 'What the hell are you doing?'

"You told me to drive without lights, Drill Sergeant.'

"'Yeah,' he said. 'But I didn't tell you to drive into a tree!'

"'But I can't see a thing,' I complained. 'What'd you think was going to happen?' Actually that part probably might have been my fault. For the most part, thinking is not an essential skill in basic training."

Ira Berkow (army, Ft. Leonard Wood, 1958) also had a memorable experience on wheels, and it involved an army vehicle's equipment that proved vital to its occupants. "We were in the middle of a convoy of about ten deuce-and-a-half (2½-ton hauling capacity) trucks going to the rifle range. There were about ten of us, and one of the guys had to pee. He really had to pee. He motioned to the lieutenant, he tried everything to get the convoy to stop, but there was no way. Finally he just couldn't wait anymore. He stood up and peed out of the back of the truck.

"And as we watched the driver of the truck behind us put on his windshield wipers."

Ladies Daze: Training Women

WHILE IT IS WELL known that President Harry Truman racially integrated the armed forces in 1948, less known is the fact that months later he signed the Women's Armed Forces Integration Act, which for the first time allowed women to serve in the military other than during wartime, and not just in a female auxiliary. More than sixty years later, with women becoming an increasingly significant portion of the armed forces and many of them suffering grievous and sometimes fatal wounds, it seems almost archaic that we had to legislate females into uniform. Still, there had been small inroads before, as during the Second World War, when women served as pilots in the Army Air Corps, ferrying newly built aircraft across the oceans to the war theaters.

In 1949, the newly founded air force welcomed four thousand women to serve mostly in medical, weather observation, photographic, and clerical positions. The first female air force recruits wore men's uniforms, complete with neckties, and in addition to physical training and military indoctrination, they also attended courses in proper posture and the use of cosmetics. As Cindy McNally (air force, Lackland, 1975) remembers, that didn't change until 1976. "When men were on the confidence course we had what was called Deportment Training. We were using the same book used in the 1950s, *How to Be a Woman in the Air Force.* In basic we were completely segregated from the men, and we attended classes which taught us essentials like how to sit like a lady, walk like a lady, put on make-up like a lady, personal hygiene, and how to avoid getting sexually transmitted diseases."

In the Marines, women had been performing clerical duties since 1918, and thousands of women serving stateside filled a variety of support roles during World War II, but it wasn't until 1949 that the Corps set up a command at Parris Island specifically to train women. In the army, the Women's Army Auxiliary Corps was created in 1942, but members had no official military status. That changed a year later when President Franklin Roosevelt signed a bill in 1943 that replaced the WAAC with the Women's Army Corps. During the Second World War, women going through basic training lived in converted stables at Ft. Des Moines and converted POW camps at several other bases, but in 1948 the first training facility created specifically for women was opened at Camp Lee, Virginia.

Females were permitted to enlist in the Navy Reserves as early as 1917. Although officially given the rank yeoman, they were known as "yeomanettes"—while women assigned to the Marine Reserves had the even more ludicrous title "Marinettes"—and they did not go through boot camp. During World War II training for the Women Accepted for Volunteer Emergency Service, the WAVES, initially took place at Iowa State Teachers' College, but in 1943 was transferred to the Bronx, New York, campus of Hunter College. Trainees were advised to bring with them "rain coat and rain hat (no umbrellas), lightweight dresses or suits, plain bathrobe, soft-soled bedroom slippers, easily laundered underwear, play suit, or shorts for physical education (no slacks), and comfortable dark brown, laced oxfords because . . . experience has proven that drilling tends to enlarge the feet."

WAVES uniforms were designed by a Parisian couturier, and as Evelyn Einfelt (navy, Lehman College, 1943) told author Curt Dalton, "We had designer clothes. The WACs had to wear green underwear! We could wear the underclothing that we liked. The WACs, everything was regulation, but we could go out and buy tailor-made uniforms that were nice."

It may seem mundane today, but the challenges of dealing with a basic training unit in which young men and women live and work together, but have to remain apart, are formidable. So it's not surprising that coeducational training stumbled initially at first, as officials demonstrated conclusively that they weren't sure how they were going to implement significant change in an organization that had not changed substantially for two hundred years.

Beginning in 1977 the army and air force began training men and women together. In 1982 the army suspended that policy, evidently because too many women were getting injured trying to keep up with the men, while the men complained that training standards had been lowered to accommodate women. The navy adopted the earlier policy in 1992 and in 1994 the army once again began mixed-gender training classes. At Lackland in 1975, Cindy McNally remembers, "Our TIs tried to pretend the men weren't there. When we marched past them our instructors would order, 'Eyes right!' or eyes left so we couldn't look at them. The only time you saw a guy was at church on Sunday, and it didn't matter if you were an atheist—every one of us went to church. Meeting a man is what a lot of women were praying for, and church was the perfect place for it. We were the most church-going people you have ever seen. We'd go a couple of times a day if possible. That was the only time we got to flirt with the guys."

Brian Deever's experience at Marine boot camp was the same. "There were women at Parris Island when I was down there in 1993," he says, "but the only time you'd see the women was at church services on Sunday. The men would sit on one side and the women across the aisle and the Drill Sergeants stayed in the middle. If we got caught looking at a woman one of the women drill instructors would warn us, 'Why are you looking at my female Marines?' Well, that was pretty obvious, wasn't it? I think the hardest part about boot camp was knowing they were there and you couldn't do anything about it."

Initially the concept of training men and women together was controversial, but as a female officer who supervised the first Army group observed, the biggest differences between male and female trainees seemed to be that "The men overloaded the washing machines because they didn't know how to use them."

Before that, Jo Dawn McEwan (army, Ft. McClellan, 1975) complained, "The guys just sent it out and it came back nice and clean, while we had to do our own damn laundry. We had three washers for an entire battalion and two of them were always broken. I'm still irritated when I think about the unfairness of it. Women definitely were treated as a problem rather than a resource."

The transition was also difficult for Drill Sergeants, who had to adjust to the changes. "We were never alone with a female recruit," says Kevin Robert Meade. "As a Drill Sergeant we have tremendous power, female recruits look up to us as a father figure, so we had to protect ourselves because without meaning to you could find yourself in a difficult situation. Perception was the key word; it wasn't necessarily what happened, but what it looked like might have happened."

The widely accepted belief about the equality of the genders notwithstanding, some trainers found that to be successful they had to motivate men and women quite differently. Chief Petty Officer Deanna Rietveld explained to a reporter the difference between motivating men and women, "You can play off a woman's emotions, asking her, 'How could you tell a mother that you killed her child because you didn't put the cotter pin in a grenade right?' She's in tears. Men are simpler. I just tell them to assume push-up position. They're stubborn and hard-headed, and that's how you motivate them."

At the heart of the early resistance to same-gender training was the assumption that because women are physically weaker than men they could not meet the same fitness standards. The objection was that relaxing the standards for females could produce an undemocratic, unfair, and dangerous system, but those differences have been mostly bridged with cleverness, leadership, discipline, and common sense. Generally men outperform women in the number of push-ups they can do, while women are often capable of doing more sit-ups. Obviously, those objections haven't been completely forgotten. "At Great Lakes," Philip Landon explained, "we were always told that the male half of a gender-integrated division was always in the best shape—because they had to do one-and-a-half-times the work."

In 1978 "Tuffy" Tofuri became one of the first male TIs to train women. "I had one thought process: They were basic recruits, and I trained them as I trained the males. The only difference was that I was not allowed in their barracks before 0600 hours, and that was the same thing with female TIs training males. The main thing I had to get accustomed to was the crying. Female recruits cried for no reason. But once you start teaching them, and they know you won't fall for their crying like their mommy and daddy did, that disappears. I would start pumping them up, telling them, 'You are no longer a child. You are a woman in the United States Air Force,' and within a few weeks they could take anything I could throw at them."

Men and women, TI Tim Price explained, "both ran the obstacle course, and they had different training standards, but they would be together for classroom work and drilling. At first it was hard for me to raise my voice to women, but all it took was getting burned once and that ended. And having previously served on the flight line and seen men and women performing the same jobs, it was not hard for me to get used to training women."

At Fort Gordon, Georgia, in 1981, one of Anthony Shaffer's Drill Sergeants was "Christine Taylor, the army's first female Drill Sergeant. The strange thing was that there wasn't anything strange about it. None of us had been through basic training before so it wasn't like we saw any difference. All we saw were her stripes. I don't remember anyone having any problem taking orders from her. I never saw or witnessed or even heard about an incident in which her authority was questioned by a trainee. She must have been about 5'2" but she definitely could ream out people. It was a great thing to watch. She was fearless. She would get right up in the face of these 6'3" guys and make them toe the line. Well, maybe not their face."

The real problem the military encounters when men and women train together, of course, is that men and women are training together. As Shaffer notes, "We had one of the first completely integrated training units, with males and females living in the same building. The results included three pregnancies and three marriages. I could never figure out where people found the time." Or the opportunity.

All of the services have instituted strict regulations designed to keep men and women apart. In theory they should not have much interest in each other, because, as a navy officer at Orlando told a reporter, "They have been hot, tired, and seen each other at their worst: the heads shaved on the guys, and no make-up on the women at three o'clock in the morning."

Everything is done to discourage attraction. For example, trainees are not permitted to wear contact lenses or their own glasses during basic training. No stylish frames. Instead they are given government-issued glasses. These dark, heavy-plastic glasses are known, and not affectionately, as "BCGs," meaning "birth control glasses," the assumption being that no member of the opposite sex could possibly find you attractive when you're wearing them.

Even so, remembered Susan Kincaid Allen (air force, Lackland, 1974), "People got busted for stupid stuff like making out in dumpsters or in the aircraft displays near the gates. They must have been some desperate eighteen-year-olds."

"You know how cold it is at Ft. Leonard Wood in February?" asked Andy McKee (army, 2008). "We were out on a field exercise, and some of the girls thought it would be fun to sneak into the guys' tents over across the no-go line. They got caught going in there by one of our Drill Sergeants, but instead of saying anything he gave them the opportunity to correct that wrong. They didn't. Instead they stayed in there and eventually sneaked back into their own tents. The next morning they got called out in front of everyone. Then he smoked the entire platoon. It was bad: weapons, PT in full gear."

Christine Knight remembers one couple getting caught in a janitorial closet at Ft. Sill in 2000. In Melissa Johnson's Ft. Sill company a male and female trainee were caught having sex in a stairwell— proving where there's a will, there's a well, or a dumpster, or tent as Drill Sergeant Kevin Robert Meade learned at Ft. Leonard Wood. "This was how desperate people got. We were out on bivouac. We had been training all day long. Everybody was tired, sweaty, and grumpy. There were no showers in the woods. So we were surprised when one recruit informed us that two trainees were hooking up. The Senior Drill Instructor went to their tent and there they were. He literally ripped off the tent and there were ten toes up and ten toes down. He looked at them and then said the most obvious words he could think of, 'Just what do you think you're doing?'

"Well, that was pretty obvious."

Survival Training: The Life You Save May Be Your Own

IN HIS SIXTH WEEK of basic Mike LaRoche was on a detail with two other trainees, loading up magazines for the firing range at Ft. Benning in 2004, when, he remembers, "Our captain came by. He just came over to me and said, 'See that Coke can behind you? Do me a favor, and can you give that to me please?' I thought that was a little odd. I didn't know why somebody left a drink sitting there, but I was not going to question it. So I grabbed it and picked it up. It started beeping really loud, a high-decibel squeal. He looked me right in the eyes and said, 'You're fucking dead.'

"I had no idea what was going on, and then he told me, 'When you get overseas the enemy will booby-trap you, and you will die. They aren't fighting us like you see in the movies. They're putting bombs in the ground. When you get to Iraq you need to be aware of everything around you at all times. I put that there when I was walking around, and you guys didn't even notice it.' At that time IEDs, Improvised Explosive Devices, were just becoming pretty common. When the captain walked away everybody wanted to know what was going down. They didn't have any idea that they were at least wounded. All they knew was that I picked up a soda can, and the next thing I was getting chewed out for being killed.

And they hadn't done anything, and they have been wounded. That was the biggest eye-opener I ever had."

While the character of the wars we fight has changed, for the most part basic training hasn't changed to meet specific challenges. The name of the enemy is always different—Chicoms, Charlie, Hajji—but little mission-specific training takes place during basic. Recruits learn the fundamentals of military life during their initial training. Their mission-specific training, their job training, takes place during the second eight weeks in AIT, or Advanced Individual Training. In AIT trainees learn how to do a specific job, their MOS, or Military Occupation Specialty. Basic training is all basic training.

LaRoche explains, "In the first few weeks of basic there was almost no mention of the wars in Iraq and Afghanistan. The one phrase that some people used was 'When you get over the pond and they are in your face . . .' Everybody knew who they were talking about.

"But after those first weeks your relationship with your Drill Sergeant begins changing. They start treating you differently; there's less yelling, less petty stuff, more emphasis on getting your work done. They begin to talk about the life after training, what our life in the military is really going to be like. Over time we developed a relationship with our superiors, and we became individuals to them rather than just a face with a number.

"We had one guy who had just returned from his deployment. I remember thinking, this guy looks like a maniac. But one day we were all sitting around eating our chow, cleaning our weapons, and he started talking to us about how it was overseas. It was just all the stuff about what we needed to watch out for. It was my first time hearing anything about it. I felt like a little kid listening to my grandfather tell a story. I remember the emotion and thinking, this dude has seen some shit. It really brought home to me why we were there."

While soldiers were in Afghanistan taking control of built-up areas, Thomas Burke was at Fort Benning, not learning the sophisticated skills he would need in deployment, like clearing buildings, but instead how to do the tasks infantrymen had always been doing. "We were still being taught how to dig foxholes for machine-gun fighting positions. The truth is that I didn't get anything out of basic that helped me with my performance; in fact, when I first got to my unit they pretty much told me to forget everything that I'd learned in basic."

Shawn Herbella's experience at Ft. Jackson in 2004 was somewhat different. "They trained us on old school stuff like digging foxholes but also some new stuff because Iraq and Afghanistan were big. They had built some mock buildings like Iraq, and we were one of the first classes to go through that training about how to clear rooms."

"Our Drill Sergeants would reference their combat experience in Iraq," Matt Farwell (army, Ft. Benning, 2005) explains. "Everything was like, 'Me shooting like this is what enabled me to kill twelve guys when I was over there.' You're like, oh shit, I'd better pay attention.

"The only thing about Iraq and Afghanistan that got incorporated was IED recognition. We were trained to look for small things out of place. An example is someone had an ammo box that they might have used as a shoeshine kit, but the drill instructor took it out of the locker and ran some wires off it. We'd walk right by it and they would tell us, 'You are now officially dead, private. Hey, private number two, please pick up your dead friend.' They tried to make us aware of our environment at all times."

Fire Men and Women: Weapons Training

E VERY TRAINEE LEARNS THIS refrain:

> This is my rifle (pointing to rifle) this is my gun (grabbing crotch); one is for shooting (pointing to rifle) and one is for fun (grabbing crotch).

This common basic training refrain dates back till at least 1942. It's a way of reminding trainees that in the military a rifle is never referred to as a "gun"; it is a rifle or a weapon. Often a recruit who made the mistake of calling it a gun would have to repeat this refrain at the top of his voice while running through the barracks holding his rifle above his head.

There was a time long ago when nearly every American was comfortable and practiced with firearms. The Second Amendment stands as a signal of how much our defense has relied on citizen-soldiers and their weapons. For many families, firearms were the necessary tools of sustenance, but as we became more urbanized there was far less need to own a weapon. While there still is quite a bit of sport shooting and hunting in this country, for basic training the military has always prudently assumed that all recruits are completely ignorant of weapons.

For every member of the military service a weapon is their most important piece of equipment. Other than in close-order drill and other mind-numbing marching exercises, the first few weeks of basic doesn't incorporate weapons training. Weapons introduced several weeks later, when there is some confidence that the trainees can follow instructions sufficiently to prevent accidents. Still, accidents happen, usually the result of foolishness, carelessness, or stupidity.

"We spent three days during our fourth week at the firing range," says Jacob Blizzard (navy, Great Lakes, 2009). "We trained with several weapons, including the M-16, a 9 mm pistol, and a 12-gauge shotgun. We did this in an enclosed facility with an instructor standing right beside us. During a live fire exercise my instructor put one shell in my shotgun for me, but then dropped another shell. There was a safety line you were never supposed to cross, and he stepped across it—right in front of the barrel of my shotgun. My shotgun was pointing right at my instructor's head and everybody started screaming at me not to move. The problem is that when people start screaming at you, the first thing you want to do is move, but I just froze. I was really scared. Later I visualized the headline, 'Navy recruit blows off head of his firearms instructor with a firearm.'"

For decades following World War II the standard-issue weapon was the M-1 Garand. It was a magnificent weapon, superbly machined, and in the right hands deadly accurate to great distances, but it was long and heavy and carried only eight rounds. During Vietnam the M-16 became the military staple, and its latest incarnation, the M-4, is short, light, and accurate for everything except sniper work. In basic, the objective is to learn how to deliver accurate aimed fire, even though in combat it is a large volume of fire and exploding projectiles that usually overwhelm the enemy. The army, air force, and Marine Corps train on the M-4, but in addition to the M-16, the navy prefers the 9 millimeter pistol and the 12-gauge shotgun, two excellent weapons for repelling boarders.

Here lies Fred/He is Dead; He didn't believe/what was said.
—**Sign on the rifle range at Ft. Bliss, Texas, 1968**

"How you gonna shoot anything when you got your eyes closed? Tell me that? How do you plan on hitting anything? Now if you want to make it and be here, and shoot like everybody else you're gonna have to open your eyes and count to five, the technique we taught you. And knock out all this emotional stuff. 'Cause I don't want you out there on my range crying and shit.

"You start crying and do what you did here, you make me scared. I'm probably scareder then you are, 'cause I'm not gonna have anybody out there being all emotional and everything 'cause you're gonna hurt somebody. Open your eyes. That weapon is not going to hurt you. That weapon has never hurt anybody, it sure ain't gonna hurt you, private. It ain't gonna hurt you one bit."
—**from the documentary** *Soldier Girls* **by Nicholas Bloomfield and Joan Churchill**

The post newspaper at Ft. Leonard Wood once pointed out, "If a trainee comes to basic expecting to shoot marksman—and fails—he probably set his sights too high!" While the goal was a marksmanship medal, basically to qualify all a recruit had to do was hit a large target. If a trainee missed the target with all of his shots he was rewarded with "Maggie's drawers," which at one time in history resulted literally in a pair of ladies' bloomers being waved.

The object of firearms training during basic is to allow troops to get comfortable handling and firing weapons. As Mike Zaleuka (army, Ft. Benning, 2009) sums it up, "You can sugarcoat it all you want, but we are learning how to kill people. What do you do at your job?"

The first time a trainee fires a weapon is always exciting—sometimes more for the people around him or her than for the trainee. A lot of them have absolutely no idea what they're doing. As Adam Mandlebaum (air force, Lackland, 1970) points out, "The night we went to the range to learn how to shoot was the one night during the whole cycle that the TIs were nice to us. When you think about it, that made a lot of sense. Why would you want to piss off someone who was holding a loaded M-16 in his hands?"

The U.S. Marine Corps Rule for Gunfighting is pretty simple: "Anything worth shooting is worth shooting twice. Ammo is cheap. Life is expensive." For some people it may be surprising to learn that the quality of military training is linked strongly to the federal budget; training troops is a complex and expensive undertaking. You would think that an item as vital as ammunition would have some kind of protection. As Jimmy Young (army, Ft. Benning, 1969) remembers, during his training he found out that was not the case: "For a couple of weeks our company ran out of money for ammunition. So instead of shooting blanks during exercises, or live rounds at the rifle range, we were instructed to shout 'Bang!' I actually got in trouble one day because instead of 'Bang!,' I yelled 'Pow!'"

"At Orlando in 1976," Kevin Johnson (navy) explains, "we only went to the firing range a couple of times. Before that, they taught us how to get the rifle from the ground to our shoulder, and then we marched to the armory, got our rifles, formed up, took the rifle from the ground, and got it up to our shoulders. Then we marched to our barracks, put our rifles in a rack, and once a week we'd pull them out and clean them. At the end we reversed the process. We only went to the firing range a couple of times. It certainly wasn't emphasized, except how you got it from the ground to your shoulder."

It was very different at Parris Island in 1969, according to Brian Dennehy. "The rifle training was real intense. We spent two weeks learning how to shoot out at the firing range. Everyone did not learn how to shoot well. I did and I became expert on the M-1."

The firing range is certainly the most dangerous part of basic training, simply because it is the firing range: live rounds are fired from high-powered rifles by inexperienced young men and women. As Gary Cooper was informed in the movie *Sergeant York*, "This is real live ammunition. A bullet hasn't got any brains. It'll hit whatever you aim at. So don't start murdering each other."

Have you ever seen an untrained person fire the rifle? This is what happens: he gets all set, gets into position, draws what he thinks is a fine bead on the target and then closes both eyes and yanks the trigger. And he wonders, why he never hit the target?

Remember this, it's instinctive, natural, for every one of us to close both eyes and tighten up when we fire a rifle . . . if we know when that rifle is going off! But when you do that you spoil your aim. You not only miss the bull's-eye but you may miss the whole target. Now there's only one way to beat nature on this proposition. That is squeeze the trigger so smoothly and to increase the pressure so steadily that you don't know when the rifle is going off. If you don't know when the rifle is going off, you can't close your eyes, flinch, spoil your aim, before the shot is fired. The worst you can do is bat your eyes after the rifle is fired and that doesn't hurt anything because the shot is already on its way.

Simple, isn't it? Now let's see exactly how you go about learning . . . trigger squeeze. . . .

> —from the U.S. Signal Corps instructional film, "Rifle Marksman Training, with the M-1," 1943

Michael Johnson, 2009 Drill Sergeant of the Year, pointed out that "There are all kinds of stories about the terrible things that have happened on the firing range, although most of them aren't true. But one afternoon we were going down range in full kit and engaging the target. Basically run and shoot. This one bone-head was running, and to this day I can't explain how it happened, he tripped and twisted his body and his weapon fired and he literally shot directly behind him—where our company commander was standing.

"Fortunately, his shot went right between our commander and the Drill Sergeant. We understood it was a mistake, but it was a serious mistake. He ended up being recycled back to day one.

It isn't always the inept trainee who is the cause of the mishap. With more than three hundred thousand trainees going through basic training every year, inevitably there will be equipment malfunctions. "I've also seen explosions in the barrel," said Johnson. "Once, I remember, this private said his weapon was swept and clear. Then he checked it. When the cold air hit the warm round, it exploded right in the Drill Sergeant's face."

Peter Flood (army, Ft. Dix, 1968) also just barely averted a serious problem at the rifle range, although it was not the fault of the equipment. "We were marching through the pine barrens to get to the firing range. There was one trainee—we called him Flipper after the dolphin—and he was somewhat challenged. We worked with him constantly on basic drills so he could get through. He was walking on the edge. When we told him to get off, he fell into the sandpit, and his weapon went muzzle-first into the sand, like a spear. He got up, pulled it out, and we kept marching. When we got to the range there was sand in the muzzle and the flash suppressor."

So far, the only adverse result was a rifle choked with sand, a problem easily fixed by disassembling the rifle and cleaning it, something the troops had already been trained to do, but that's not what this soldier did. "What he did was he pulled off one of his bootlaces and tied it to a handkerchief, then ran the shoelace down the barrel of his weapon into the breach and tried to pull the whole handkerchief through. Apparently the handkerchief got stuck in the barrel.

"When we got to the range everybody took their firing positions. Then I looked down the firing line I saw all the barrels pointing down range, and there was one that looked like a joke gun, with a flag hanging out of it. The Drill Sergeants started calling that all was clear to fire, but I screamed that we were not clear. Had he pulled that handkerchief down to the chamber and tried to clean that weapon, it probably would have exploded. This kid really didn't grasp how close he was to hurting himself, and maybe others."

Most military weapons are automatic or semi-automatic, meaning the spent cartridge is ejected from the right side of the rifle after each shot. "I had never fired a weapon, but it turned out that my left eye is much stronger than my right eye," Norman Batansky (army, Ft. Jackson, 1969) explains. "So I had to fire as a lefty, but I didn't have the slightest idea how the shell came out of the weapon. They didn't bother explaining that to us. So when I fired for the first time it came out hot, hit me right in the neck, and burned a scar right there."

"We always had troops with what we called 'M-1 eye,'" James Vaughn (army, Ft. Jackson/Ft. Gordon, 1962) recalls. "They didn't know how to hold the rifle correctly and hadn't been warned about the recoil, so when they fired their weapon their thumb was too close to their eye, it hit them in the eye giving them a black eye. You could always tell when a company had been to the firing range by the number of black eyes you saw."

Ira Berkow (army, Ft. Leonard Wood, 1958) also had never fired a rifle, but assumed that it was simple: "I thought you just aimed and fired, how hard could that be, but then they started teaching us the various different firing positions. There was a prone position, a kneeling position, a position where you had the rifle resting on a ledge, and then there was the squatting position. That was the position I couldn't do, I just couldn't do it. I was athletic, but I couldn't do this. If I was forced to shoot at the enemy from a squatting position I would have shot myself in the head."

Val Nicholas (army, Fort Ord, 1974) remembers how he learned to shoot. "They taught us a mantra that we had to repeat over and over: 'Breathe, relax, aim, and squeeze.' Then to make sure we weren't afraid of the M-16's recoil, first they made us hold the butt against our forehead and fire it, and then after we did that, they made us hold it against our crotch and empty the clip.

"In all honesty, there were some people who really liked that."

Nicholas trained at Fort Ord, California, which is located on beautiful Monterey Bay. "Our firing ranges were on the ocean, and every once in a while a whale would come into the bay, and I don't care what we were supposed to be shooting at, everyone started unloading their clips out to sea. One time a deer walked behind the range. That was probably the dumbest deer in deer history, walking into a firing range. It had no chance. Before the range master could tell us to stop, it was done."

Myth #4: Death on the Infiltration Course

Among the most memorable nights during basic is the Night Infiltration Course (NIC), which has now become known as "Nick at Night." Of all the aspects of basic, the live fire crawl has changed the least through the decades. In this exercise, trainees have to cradle their rifles and crawl across a field in the dark and under barbed wire, while machine guns fire live ammunition a few feet above their heads. The purpose of the live-fire training is not to teach bad tactics—on a battlefield enemy machine guns covering a barbed wire obstacle would be shooting directly at the troops, and most of them would become casualties—but rather to instill confidence. The excitement generated by engaging in something new, thrilling, and supposedly dangerous is very high, and success in completing it has a strong impact on a trainee. In fact, there may be no better way to encourage people to crawl low and fast than firing a searing stream of live ammunition a few feet over their head.

Without doubt, trainees will be warned that if they stand up during this exercise they could be killed—and that in a previous cycle a trainee did exactly that and was cut down by the machine guns. There may well have been some isolated incidences in the history of trainees standing up during this exercise, but certainly it is very rare. Here's the question: People are firing machine guns directly over your head. Why would you want to stand up?

Melissa Johnson (army, Ft. Sill, 2001) admits, "I definitely was scared when they started firing live rounds. I wanted to get up and run—but then I realized, wow, that's a seriously bad idea. Instead, I just had to slow down and remind myself I could get through it if I focused on what I was doing."

When Ralph Strauss did his crawl at Ft. Knox in 1945, the cadre evidently had too much time on its hands, because its members viewed it as an entertainment. "You knew they were live bullets because every fourth bullet was a tracer, and you could see it. You crawled with the muzzle of your rifle higher so you wouldn't get it dirty, but what was strange was that there was a bridge over this field, and the officers and their wives and sweethearts were standing there watching us crawl."

At Ft. Leonard Wood, even after a passage of more than twenty years, almost nothing had changed. As Roger Hayes wrote his Vietnam memoir *On Point,* "The live fire exercise was one of the highlights of basic training. Two M-60 machine guns were positioned on one edge of the range . . . and fired continuously as we crawled the range. . . . "Paths had been formed where trainees from other companies had crawled. It was easiest to follow these trails and low spots underneath the wire. Unfortunately, it had rained recently and these indentations were filled with water.

"As we concluded the course, we were allowed to stand behind the machine guns and watch as our fellow trainees followed us. I was surprised to see that steel bars had been placed parallel to the ground under the barrel of each gun. This was to prevent the machinegunner from accidentally shooting any of us. In a way, it was a disappointment. We had believed this was a life-threatening exercise."

Of course, the Drill Sergeants had their own way of dealing with that. Before Troy Bayse's (army, Ft. Benning, 2010) platoon went through the course "they told us that it had been closed down for a while just before we got there because during one of those exercises one of the turret safety mounts that prevent the weapon from aiming down broke, and the barrel went down and some guys ended up getting killed."

At Parris Island, Marine recruits in 1980 crawled through the same course, although as Thomas Kilbride discovered, it wasn't actually very dangerous. "They watered down the dirt into mud, and the barbed wire was about eight inches off the ground, and you had to crawl under it without getting mud in your rifle. They also have trip flares that will go off if you hit them, but it's real for you, you're filthy and tired and you're not used to crawling like that, and then you get punished for not finishing on time."

As Carl Burgess (army, Ft. Jackson, 2006) describes his experience, while the nature of war has changed, the weapons that are commonly used have changed, and certainly the terrain has changed, Nick at Night has remained essentially the same. "As the first wave crested, the real machine guns opened up. You could hear the low thump, thump, thump of the .50 caliber machine gun. A flare went up in the air and the entire field was illuminated. We were ordered over the wall. I clambered over the wall into the sand and began crawling. There were dozens of people in front of me with trails behind where they had crawled.

"I crawled forward about twenty-five meters and came to some barbed wire. I turned on my back and shimmied under it. On my back I could clearly see the reddish orange tracer rounds from the guns zipping overhead. Even though I knew they were over ten feet above me, they sure looked awfully close."

Burgess passed one female who was on the verge of panicking, screaming, "I can't breathe!" He glanced at her and saw that she was fine. Then he told her, "'Stop, just take a couple deep breaths and keep going.' She did and I pushed on. About halfway through I began thinking, this is fun but I was expecting more realism.

"The last ten meters were the worst. I was getting tired and wasn't making progress very quickly, I felt like I was standing still. I was covered front to back in wet sand. There are Drill Sergeants standing at the finish line, letting you know if you were done and it was safe to stand up. I finished in the first third of my platoon."

In addition to how to fire a rifle, recruits are taught how to use an array of other weapons:

Sergeant: "Let us take a look at the claymore mine and see exactly what it looks like. The weapon's primary uses are defensive in nature. It's the United States Army's primary ambush initiating weapon. . . . The mine right now is responsible for approximately 8 percent of all casualties for such a small weapon. The weapon is directional in nature, that is, whatever way you set the device up and set it off, the blast from the weapon will travel along the ground in that direction. For this reason you have got to always face the weapon toward the enemy or away from friendly troops. There's enough C-4 in the back of this mine, if you were to take it all out and roll it up, it would be about the size of a baseball. If I were to plug a blasting cap into it, and place it right in front of me, and set it off, it would kill just about everybody in the bleachers . . .

"You'll notice that in the front of the mine, you have got several hundred steel ball bearings embedded in molded plastic. I can see from the looks on your faces that you're starting to get the picture. You place these ball bearings in the front, you place the C-4 behind it, you put the back on, and because the mine is curved the way it is, when you set the device off, it will act as a giant shotgun.

It will propel these pellets to the front, approximately two hundred and fifty meters on a fan of sixty degrees. That is one sixth of a circle."

—from the documentary *Basic Training* by Fred Wiseman

Trainees also learn how to throw a live hand grenade, which is arguably one of the most dangerous—and exciting—days of the cycle. As Homer Hickam (army, Ft. Leonard Wood, 1966) discovered, the potential for serious injury is very real. "I actually witnessed a live grenade going in the wrong direction. Our Drill Sergeant had showed us over and over and over how to pull the pin then throw the grenade. We were standing in line and one of the guys about three revetments down from me pulled the pin—and dropped his grenade right there. Nobody had the presence of mind to yell 'Live grenade,' instead they just took off running. We didn't know exactly what was going on, but everybody started ducking. Fortunately, each revetment was surrounded by sandbags, so the only damage he did was to blow up a lot of sandbags."

At Ft. Jackson in 2010 Tynesha Brown had her own near miss, "For safety reasons we lined up behind a door leading to a pillbox set-up. They put the grenade in your hand, opened the door, and you went out and pulled the pin and threw your grenade. For everyone before me our Drill Sergeant opened the door and pushed them out. I was so excited that he didn't have to do that for me. Soon as the door opened I ran out full speed—and tripped. I fell right on top of my grenade. Fortunately I hadn't pulled the pin so there was no real danger. But as I lay there, the only thought going my head was, 'Shit, now he's going to be mad.' I heard him shout in the background, 'Brown. Get up!' I looked at him and said right back, 'What? D'you think I was gonna take a nap?'

"Listen Up You Mens":
Speaking Military

IN MARINE BOOT CAMP when a Drill Instructor wants recruits to "listen up," or pay particular attention to what that he is saying, he'll command "Ears." In response, recruits will shout "Open, Sir," which means they are listening. Similarly, when a DI wants them to stop whatever they're doing and look at him, he'll command, "Eyeballs," to which recruits will respond, "Click, Sir."

The ability to follow commands without hesitation or question is at the core of military order—and may well be the primary lesson learned in basic training. All training is a continuing exercise in the value of clear and concise communication, although admittedly sometimes that means very loud communication. A lot of trainees never forget the most memorable observations uttered by drill instructors. It would seem impossible to succeed in basic training without speaking even a little Drill Instructor English—but Philip Landon (navy, Great Lakes, 2005) conducted his own unique experiment in boot camp: Is it possible to get through eight weeks of training without understanding English? "My bunkmate was a Puerto Rican kid named Torres, Torres, Torres. When I found out he spoke only a few words of English, I decided to try to help him get through it. My Spanish was limited but functional. I helped him with everything, from making our bed to drilling, and he was always next to me. And that was encouraged in the military because they want you to buddy-up with your bunkmate.

"We got into the fourth week before they found out he didn't speak English. They caught him because all he said was 'Yes, Sir!' over and over, whatever the question or order was: 'Yes, Sir! Yes, Sir!' They had this exercise where they'd have us step through our skivvies all the time and he stepped through his upside down. They kept calling him an idiot, and in response he smiled and said, 'Yes, Sir!'"

Philip's father, Daniel Landon, told this story in his comic play, *Basic Training*:

MASTER CHIEF: Did you have any indication over the last three weeks that Recruit Bronx (Torres) had any problems with language?

(RECRUIT TRAINER) KOWALSKI: No, Chief. He's just timid, or stupid, or both.

CHIEF: Very well. Issue an order.

KOWALSKI: Recruit Bronx drop and give me twenty. (TORRES remains at attention) Run in place. (TORRES nervously looks at MASTER CHIEF THOMPSON and LANDON) Don't look at him. Name the president of the country.

TORRES: El presidente es . . . Vincente Fox!

KOWALSKI: No, stupid, the American President.

TORRES: No habla English.

KOWALSKI: Bush, stupid. George Bush! He's out! He's out right now! Him, too! Recruit Jersey (LANDON) has been playing us all along.

MASTER CHIEF: You want to go to the Captain and explain

how it took us three weeks to find out one of our recruits couldn't speak any fucking English at all? You want to do that, Petty Officer, and have us both back driving truck routes to Baghdad by Easter?

"Smoke 'Em If You Got 'Em": The Military and Tobacco

THE SMOKING LAMP HAS now been extinguished—forever. For many recruits the most difficult adjustment in basic training is giving up tobacco. Tobacco in any form—cigarettes, cigars, chew—is prohibited, and all tobacco products are considered contraband and confiscated the first week. This is ironic, considering that the military may be responsible for creating countless smokers. Years ago, almost all trainees smoked cigarettes, and if they hadn't smoked before they entered the service, they started soon after enlistment. Smoking was so pervasive that each C-Ration meal contained a pack of four cigarettes, usually the unfiltered kind, thus delivering the maximum amount of addictive tobacco. In civilian life a significant percentage of the price of cigarettes is tax, but post and base exchanges, which are federal enterprises, were free of tax, and as late as 1967 a carton consisting of ten packs—two hundred cigarettes—cost two dollars. The barracks usually had sand-filled fire cans at either end for people to extinguish their cigarettes. At Ft. Sill, Oklahoma, in 1943, according to Jerry Leitner, "The whole attitude toward cigarettes was 'Smoke 'em if you got 'em.' Everybody smoked. Cigarettes were a dime a pack. And we would take a ten-minute smoke break every hour—because the sergeants needed to have a cigarette as much as we did."

Cigarettes were an important part of the military culture. Journalist Ralph Turtinan (Marines, Parris Island, 1945) reported that as part of a hazing ritual a recruit was forced to "puff on a half-dozen cigarettes simultaneously with a bucket over his head."

"Everybody in the military smoked in the 1970s," explained Cindy McNally. "We'd be standing in formation, and the drill instructor would bark out, 'Smoke 'em if you got 'em.' I didn't smoke when I got to Lackland, but the second time she gave that command I found myself a pack of cigarettes, because it was the only time we weren't standing at parade rest or attention. You got wise pretty fast that if you smoked you could get a break and talk to everybody. So I started smoking."

And not just cigarettes, at least not at Lackland. According to Susan Kincaid Allen, "The girl who had the cot next to me was a cowgirl from Montana who dipped snuff. When they started letting us smoke after the first few weeks, they didn't give her snuff back until we all got together and complained that it was a double standard." She got her snuff.

Smokers had to field strip their "coffin nails." Jerry Leitner recalls, "The first thing they taught us was how to field strip a cigarette. If you got caught throwing down a cigarette butt there definitely was some discipline involved. So you learned how to cut a butt open with a thumbnail and scatter the ashes and tobacco in the wind, then roll the remaining paper into a little ball."

Obviously not everybody bothered to field strip their cigarettes, instead they just tossed away butts and filters. The result was a regular police call, in which recruits had to clean up an entire area. "They were tough about that at Ft. Dix," Saul Wolfe says. "The sergeant would tell us, 'I don't want to see anything but asses and elbows,' meaning we'd better be bent over picking up everything on the ground."

Jo Dawn McEwan (army, Ft. McClellan, 1975) learned that lesson so well that more than two decades after leaving the service "I'll put my butt in my pocket or purse, the one thing I won't do is drop it on the ground. I picked up too many cigarettes in my time."

"We were pretty hard on people who threw down butts at Parris Island," Dwayne Duckworth (Marines, 1948) recalls. "We had a smoking lamp, which meant people were allowed to smoke at a certain time. When they tried to catch a smoke at other times we had problems. When I was an instructor my junior sergeant caught one of the recruits smoking behind a hut. When he got caught he tried to throw away the butt. Our Drill Instructor was furious. So he ordered us to hold a complete funeral service for that butt. That recruit had to dig a hole six feet deep and three feet wide for that butt, which was buried in it."

A Dream Job: The Recruit
Never Sleeps

AMONG THE VARIOUS SKILLS that many people take away from basic training is how to sleep standing up with their eyes wide open. It's an art form that has to be learned, and the military provides plenty of opportunity to learn it. Although trainees are supposed to get eight hours of sleep per night, less the hour they spend on fire watch, the reality is usually very different, especially at the beginning of the training cycle. Sleep deprivation is an important tool used during basic to remind trainees they're not at home any more. Steven Singer (army, Ft. Polk, 1970) may well have summed it up for everybody who has ever been to basic when he admitted, "I personally didn't care for the hours of the job. I'm not a morning guy. For me to get started with my day at 4:00 A.M. took me a little while to get used to.

"The barracks at Ft. Dix were the same barracks they had been using since the 1930s," Dan Blatt (army, Ft. Dix, 1962) remembers. "They were fire traps. So we had people alternating fire watch duty all night. You'd do it for two hours, which was basically half of your sleep. You'd walk around listening to people dreaming out loud. Then we would be up and standing in formation, in subzero weather, at 5:00 in the morning. Then they would run us for an hour until we worked up a sweat. We were exhausted, and we were freezing—and that's when they would tell us to sing."

The plethora of training objectives, restrictions, and rules made certain that some of them were counterproductive or even mutually exclusive. According to Tom Mellor, at Ft. Benning in 1999, "For some weird reason they weren't allowed to put the lights on till 5:00 A.M., but we had to be outside by 5:30. With all the things we needed to get done we had to be up at 4:45 so we ended up having to do all our work in the dark. I never could figure out who we were trying to hide from. It was kind of a game."

"We were always tired," says Herb Cohn (army, Ft. Dix, 1963). "We would do anything to get a few extra minutes sleep. That was the one thing I usually got in trouble for, sneaking off somewhere to take a nap. The thing you learn is where the best places to hide are, and usually it was in the grass somewhere, behind a tree. It was really hard to grab a nap in the bunks, or under the bunk, which was a favorite spot, because periodically they would come through looking for people sleeping. And a lot of time they would find them."

"I was lucky," explains Jack Fut (army, Ft. Dix, 1962). "I had guard duty at midnight, and I was up in a tower and I fell asleep on my feet. One of the guards would come around to check and suddenly a loud voice woke me up by asking, 'Fut, are you asleep?' How was I going to answer that question, 'Not anymore?' That's a court-martial offense, I think. 'No, Sir!' I snapped."

Kahlil Ashanti (air force, Lackland, 1992) had to stay up all night on dorm guard duty. "I thought I could do it. I can remember standing there at attention and waking up when my nose hit the floor. I literally fell asleep on my feet and fell straight down on my nose. I thought I'd broken it. At the same time, admittedly it was pretty comfortable lying there on the floor and I did get almost eight seconds sleep on the way down."

There is one thing guaranteed about basic training: Basic training definitely is a cure for insomnia. After a full day of training the problem is staying awake, not falling asleep. "Everybody was always exhausted," Paul Setmaer (air force, Lackland, 1977) says firmly. "You could see the effect that stress had on people in the barracks at night. For a lot of people, that stress manifested itself by sleepwalking or reacting to some kind of stimulus in their sleep. Every once in a while I'd pull CQ, charge of quarters, basically a dorm guard, which meant I'd have to spend a couple of hours patrolling the dorm. All that meant was you walked back and forth amongst everybody else who was sleeping to make sure that nothing illicit was going on. But every once in a while somebody would be sleepwalking, and I'd have to wake them up, or as I walked past a bunk that person would detect the movement and literally leap up. They were so wound up they'd sit up and start talking in their sleep.

"We had one guy who had a classic term that he said to people if they said something stupid: 'What are you, effin' wild?' It was funny when he said it. But one night when I was on CQ he actually sat up, grabbed his boots, and yelled, 'What are you, effin' wild?,' and hurled the boots into his metal locker, which woke up everybody else, and a lot of them figured it was time to get up so they climbed out of their bunks, while he laid down and went right back to sleep having absolutely no idea what he'd done."

TI Price had one recruit who would wake in the night from a regular nightmare. "He constantly had these dreams that he was waking up inside a coffin, in the ground with the worms eating him. It must have been terrifying because his eyes would be bulging out of his head and he would be covered with sweat from head to toe. To him, this was real."

While sleepwalking doesn't seem like a serious problem, in the navy it can be cause for dismissal from the service. "You can't have sleepwalkers on a ship," points out Holly Kale (navy, Great Lakes, 2003). "In boot camp I had a sleepwalker in my division. We were sleeping in bunk beds, which were real close together, and one night she woke up and tried to sit up really fast. She slammed her head on the bottom of the upper bunk and knocked herself out. She had to go to medical and we never saw her again."

Maybe the worst thing a recruit could do in basic was deprive anyone else of sleep—as Tom Mellor learned at Ft. Benning in 1999. "One night I really needed to make a call," he said. "So I snuck into the reception area and got caught. Okay, I figured whatever they did to me I could take it. But what the Drill Sergeant did was wake up the whole bay at one o'clock in the morning for PT and pointed out that the only reason they were up and out there was because I felt a need to make a phone call. Okay, I thought, I'm definitely a dead man."

It was difficult to alleviate the stress of training, but practical jokes were an occasional outlet. Some trainees are natural jokers, while others are natural marks, but if you weren't the mark, most people usually thought that the joke was at least worth a little smile.

One of the most annoying jokers of all time was in Brian Deever's platoon at Parris Island in 1993. "For some reason this guy thought it was funny to play practical jokes in the middle of the night. Here's a really bad combination: a practical joker with a pocket full of firecrackers walking guard duty in a barracks full of stressed out Marine recruits fast asleep in the middle of the night. Somehow this guy got hold of some fireworks. I have no idea how he got them, but when he was on fire watch he decided to set off the fireworks—in a garbage can. Maybe he forgot that our Drill Instructors slept there, too."

If this idiot couldn't guess that it's a bad idea to wake up DIs in the middle of the night, he learned it that evening, because the entire platoon got punished for it. "That was the DIs' way of reminding us that it's one team, one fight in the Marine Corps. This is why we were outside crawling around in the sand pits at 2:00 A.M."

Thought for Food:
Military Chow

Camp Sherman has a completely equipped refrigeration and ice making plant, which assures the boys that their food will be kept in perfect condition. Every meat is inspected by government inspectors. One of the most highly specialized and efficient camp organizations is the "Department of Eats." By nightfall the young fellow from back home forgets all about his languid gait and dyspeptic pallor and treats his cavernous inner self to generous heaps of honest-to-goodness body building food.

—World War I army film: *Basic Training at Camp Sherman*

PFC ELVIS PRESLEY (ARMY, Ft. Hood, 1958) once said, "After a hard day of basic training, you could eat a rattlesnake." Apparently the military was listening.

As anyone who has enjoyed the fine cuisine served to recruits during basic training will attest, there is nothing better than military chow. Absolutely nothing. That's not a compliment: Many recruits report that eating nothing was often better than what they were served, but of course they say that well after the fact. For decades, military dining establishments were called "mess halls," and quite properly so in many cases. Before compartmented trays, the food was piled unceremoniously one item atop the previous one, and dinner grew before one's eyes into a large, undifferentiated lump of wilted lettuce, watery mashed potatoes, sliced gray mystery meat, congealed gravy, limp broccoli, and cherry Jell-O with the density of concrete. Meals were not meant to be enjoyed but were designed instead merely to provide nourishment, without any of the sensory appeal of actual food.

Instead of "mess hall," trainees now eat in a "dining facility," cooks are "food service technicians," and the haphazard pile of stuff on a plate is now "food."

Since chow time is at a premium, the goal is to feed as many people as rapidly as possible. Drill Instructors at Parris Island referred to meals as "Eat. Duck," meaning: duck in, duck out, and eat at attention. Army Drill Sergeants ordered their troops to "Swallow now, chew later."

According to Val Nicholas, Drill Sergeants at Ft. Ord "had a competition to determine who could move his entire platoon through the mess hall the fastest, and so I never actually sat down to eat. I never saw the food for more than a few seconds, because, once we got it on the tray we had to eat it before we got to the table, and then get the hell out of the mess hall. One of the rules that they strictly enforced was that whatever food you took you had to eat. So there were times to get out of the mess hall we were eating everybody else's meals."

"I remember that there was a sign outside the chow hall," Robert Oxford (navy, Great Lakes, 1965–66) explains, " 'Take all you want, but eat all you take.' "

Doug Kasunic remembers that same sign hanging outside the chow hall in San Diego in 1963. "They didn't care if you ate one scrambled egg or fifty, but if you took fifty you'd better eat all fifty.

You couldn't take fifty and leave two on your plate. If you did you definitely had a problem. I went to boot camp as a little scrawny kid weighing 116 pounds, and when I came out of there nine weeks later I was a muscular 145 pounds."

How Marines eat, according to an unidentified Drill Instructor in a 1960s Official U.S. Marine Corps video:

"I'm gonna run you in in two lines. You will join the chow line. You will take one tray per man. The next thing you will see are bins. In these bins are knives, forks, and spoons. Each man will take one knife, one fork, and one spoon, which you will put in your right hand. You will hold a tray with both hands. The next thing you will see will be a cup. You'll put it in your left hand. You will not talk. You will march straight in, and when you reach the end of the line, you will go to a table. Six men to a table. When you go to that table, you will all stand up until that table is filled up. Then the last man at the table will say, 'Ready. Seat.' When you go into a chow hall you will eat everything you take. When you are through eating you will go to the rear of the mess hall. You will eat and get out of this mess hall, and you will not sit inside and talk. Soon as you are outside, you will get in formation at a position of attention until your Drill Instructor gets outside. Is that clear?"

The rules of basic etiquette were similar at Lackland, according to Cindy McNally. "We had what we called square meals. The first person to get to the table stood at attention and remained at attention with her tray in front of her until there were four people at the table, and then we all sat at the same time. The square meal meant taking your fork, getting your food, and then bringing it up to your mouth at right angles—and do it in two minutes or less."

Although many people thought the food was awful, some found it good, even deliciously like home. "I loved it," Ben Currin (army, Ft. Bragg, 1968) says. "I'd hear people complaining about army chow.

I came from a small hometown, and we didn't have any fancy restaurants, just cooked meals on the table, so like a lot of people what we ate in the mess halls wasn't that much different from what I ate at home. You had your meat, vegetables, potato, your milk, tea, and coffee. There were a few items I did eat for the first time, one of them being what was called S.O.S."

A staple of military chow halls is the infamous chopped beef on white toast, better known as "shit on a shingle," "same old stuff," or on occasion, simply, mystery meat. In polite company, it's S.O.S. In military recipe books, it is called "Creamed Chipped Beef on Toast," and it resembles nothing so much as Southern sausage and biscuit gravy—except without the sausage or biscuit.

Chef Noah H. Belew, who joined the Marines in the early 1940s, provided the recipe:

Ingredients
1½ pounds extra lean hamburger or ground chuck
2 tablespoons butter or oleo
1 cup chopped onion
3 tablespoons flour
2 tablespoons granulated garlic
2 tablespoons soy sauce (or less to taste)
1 tablespoon Worcestershire sauce
2 cups milk
salt and pepper to taste

Directions
Brown meat, add butter, and stir. Add onions and cook until you can see through them. Add flour, stir and cook two or three minutes. Add garlic, soy sauce, Worcestershire

sauce, salt and pepper. Mix thoroughly. Add milk and stir until thickens. Serve over toast or biscuit.

Actually, the basis of the mystery sauce with which the meat is covered is the classic French sauce, Bechamel, and it should be somewhat suggestive of sage, the dominant herb in sausage, and have the strong bite of black pepper. It almost cries for the eater to add a generous amount of hot sauce, which the real S.O.S. aficionado will do. Originally, the dish was made with thinly sliced dried beef, but as that is now prohibitively expensive, ground beef is the protein ingredient.

Traditionally, there were no choices. This was the armed forces, and a mess hall was not intended to be Les Loges de l'Aubergade. A trainee ate what was offered, and if he didn't like it, he ate nothing. There was food, even if it was not particularly appetizing, and if you were hungry, it was your own fault. Years ago there undoubtedly were committed vegetarians in uniform, and so either their intense hunger was overwhelming and they, too, ate the mystery meat, or they ate only the mashed turnips. As a matter of fact, since the vegetables were probably prepared with lard, they were loath to eat even the turnips. Today, there is usually a whole garden of vegetables available, and so you can be both in uniform and a vegetarian. As Michael Volkin (army, Ft. Leonard Wood, 2001) reports, "Even in the field the army offers vegetarian MREs, Meals Ready to Eat," and recently the armed forces began offering a healthier menu at training bases, including more vegetables and less fried food, with milk substituted for soda.

The Weight Is Worth It:
The Miracle of Military Meals

W HAT IS KNOWN ABOUT chow in training is that it has the ability to perform miracles. When it is combined in large doses with exercise and activity, people who need to gain weight, gain weight, and incredibly, people who need to lose weight, lose weight. As former TI Mike Harrel marvels, "It still baffles me. When I took my physical I had to eat a bunch of bananas and drink a lot of water to make the minimum weight standards. I was 122 pounds soaking wet. Five weeks later I graduated from basic and weighed 150 pounds. When you go into basic you're eating three meals a day and exercising regularly and going to bed at a specific time. That program would change people. It's the miracle of basic training."

It certainly changed the life of baseball Hall of Famer Tom Seaver (Marines, San Diego, 1962). Seaver joined when he was seventeen years old, "and I was about 5'9", 160 pounds. At the end of the next eighteen months, including the time I spent at boot camp, I was 6'1", 205 pounds. I was solid, and so obviously the Marine Corps played a large role during my growth spurt."

Congressional Medal of Honor recipient Sammy Lee Davis grew an inch—although he does not credit the army for that—and added twenty-five pounds in training. Val Nicholas was 5'9" and

130 pounds when he entered basic, "A stick, but when I got to the army, within twelve weeks, including my advance training, I went up to 160 pounds of muscle. I noticed at the same time that people who came in overweight came down, and at the end we all looked the same. They talk about Jenny Craig and all these weird diets, but whatever your weight issue, if you really want to get into shape then go to basic training."

"Before I joined the army I did a lot of triathlons and marathons," says Matt Riker (army, Ft. Benning, 2005). "I'm 6'5" and maybe I weighed 170 pounds. I was skinny, but the food wasn't so bad, and I ate a lot of it. And it worked out real well. Anytime I finished everything I had, other people would give me whatever they didn't want to eat. I ended up putting on about twenty-five pounds."

Dwayne Duckworth (Marines, San Diego, 1948) had precisely the same experience when he went through training. "I was so thin when I went in, that my Drill Instructor said, 'If they ask you if you're getting enough food to eat, tell them no.' One day our general inspected my rifle and asked me if I was getting enough to eat and I said firmly, 'No, Sir!' The general asked me how much I weighed when I came to San Diego. I said, 'About 130 pounds, Sir.' Then he asked me what I weighed at that time, 'About 160 pounds, Sir.'

"He smiled and said firmly, 'Private, you are getting enough to eat.'"

Everything about basic training was designed for people to get in the best possible shape and reach their optimal weight. As Mike Volkin points out, "I wanted to start the day with a big hot breakfast. The army wanted me to start it with push-ups."

With exercise part of every day, it's almost impossible for overweight people not to lose weight. Joe Lisi (Marines, Parris Island, 1969) weighed 196 when he went in. "I was called a Fat Body," he explains. "That meant when I got on the chow line I had to announce loudly to each server, 'Fat body!' That meant that they wouldn't give me a full portion of food or cake. I only got the healthy stuff, but as a result in eight weeks I lost forty-six pounds."

Tom Mellor was overweight when he began training at Ft. Benning in 1999. "They would pick on the overweight people at first, but if they saw you were trying they would leave you alone. It was those people who didn't give any effort who suffered. The cooks would make desserts in the mess hall, but only the sergeants were allowed to eat it. The leftovers got thrown in the trash out in the back. There were some people who were always hungry; no matter how much they ate, they were always looking for food. So the Dumpster was like a banquet hall for them. We did have some kids who would go Dumpster diving for cake. The sergeants caught them doing this, so what they did to punish them was put a desk in front of the formation, load up a plate with junk, and give the person who got caught three minutes to finish everything on that plate.

"Everybody knew what was coming next: After the recruit finished eating the Drill Sergeants would work him out in front of the platoon until all that food came up. It was really disgusting, but it definitely made the point."

On many bases just getting into the mess hall required performing some physical activity. On some bases trainees have to do at least ten pull-ups or a set or two on the horizontal ladder before being allowed into the chow hall. Both exercises consisted of hauling your entire weight against the pull of gravity. People who are out of shape are generally not very strong, so having to do pull-ups or cross the horizontal ladder is a test of enormous strength and will. If a trainee is overweight, he won't get much to eat until he loses enough weight to perform the required entrance exercise. "I weighed 245 pounds," explains Eric Segal (army, Ft. Dix, 1965). "When we were going through the line getting our uniforms I asked them, 'What have you got in a jumbo?' Before we went into the mess hall we were required to do a minimum of fifteen bars on the horizontal ladder. Me, support my weight for fifteen bars? You kidding me? But it was either figure out a way to do that or starve. The rule was you were allowed to drop off once, and so I learned to pace myself. There were eight bars across, and somehow I'd manage to do eight, then drop off, then come back with the seven I needed. By the end of basic I'd dropped more than thirty pounds."

"You had to do the horizontal ladder two times before they'd let you into the mess hall," according to Paul Steingruby III (army, Ft. Jackson, 1978). "If you couldn't do two of them you'd be out there on the ground doing push-ups and eating off a plate, but if you finished in the top group, they would let you sit and talk in the mess hall.

"The thing was that even when we thought we were getting away with something the Drill Sergeants knew everything that was going on. In the mess hall there was an ice cream cooler right next to the milk dispenser, and everyone was allowed to grab an ice-cream bar as we went out. Usually we were permitted to go directly back to our barracks. But some guys would grab five and six Dreamsicles and put them in their shirts or in their pants pockets as they ran outside, and then when we got to the barracks we'd split them up. For several weeks nobody got caught. But then one very hot day in September we ran outside—and our Drill Sergeants were standing there waiting for us. And they were smiling. Smiling Drill Sergeants is a bad sign. We formed up, and for a half hour they had us doing every type of drill: running in place, rolling around on the ground, endless sit-ups and push-ups. And you could see those melting, squashed Dreamsicles oozing out of every pocket. Practically every uniform was stained vanilla and orange, and no one said one word about it. It was a perfect basic training experience—it was completely hysterical, everybody knew it, but not one person laughed."

Body Building: The Shape of Recruits to Come

MANY YOUNG PEOPLE ENTER military service just as their lives are changing dramatically. These are formative years. They are getting taller, stronger, and more mature. They are learning an enormous number of life lessons, lessons that will stay with them for the rest of their lives, and when they emerge from basic, they are entirely different people than they were when they began the process. They are changing from children into adults, and they are doing it over a very short period of time. Everything that they do, and everything that happens to them, is magnified by the lens of maturation.

Dennis Stead, who may have spent the longest period of time as a trainee in the history of Parris Island, understands the great changes that are wrought by being a young adult in military service. When he enlisted in 1960 he was 6'1" tall and was about 265 pounds. "I was always fat," he said. "When I was fourteen years old I weighed 270 pounds. When I got to Parris Island my DI went crazy on me, words I can't even describe. The first week the best I could do was only *two* push-ups. Instead of taking it out on me, he took it out on the rest of the platoon. 'Oh, Private Stead, you can't do five push-ups? Tell you what you're going to do. Private Stead is so tired he's just going to lay there and rest while all of you are going to do twenty because Private Stead can't do three.' Now eighty-five guys hated my guts, and it was only the first week. There aren't many better incentives to improve than that."

Because he was highly motivated, Stead made steady progress. He was large and lumbering and still out of shape, but he had good stamina, and given enough time and support, he was determined to complete boot camp. "But after a couple of weeks I got mononucleosis and spent a month in the hospital. Eventually, they put me in what was called a Strength Platoon, a fat man's platoon. That's where all hell broke loose because those guys were serious about me losing weight and gaining strength.

"The deal in that platoon was they were either going to make you or break you. Either you would work hard enough to change your life forever, or you would be out. It was the beginning of summer, and it was hot and in the morning they would wake us up and make us put on heavy clothes, including our sweatshirts and winter jackets, then pull the hood up and tie the drawstrings tight around our necks so we'd sweat. Each morning they marched us down to an old closed-down barracks. I'll never forget it. My life changed in that room. Everything had been sealed. It was very long, very dark, and very, very hot. And then they would start running us."

The cadre was always on the verge of turning the entire unit into victims of heat stroke. "We just kept running in a huge oval, the full length of the barracks, and then back up again. Sweating horribly. Suddenly I saw white spots in front of my eyes. I tried to keep going, I wouldn't quit, and the next thing I knew I was laying on the ground outside. I had run the full length of the building, and run right through the wall. I took out the entire window casing, all the wood, all the glass, everything. I had absolutely no memory of it, I'd blacked out and kept running. 'You're going to live,' they told me, but that was the end of training for that day.

"The next day we came back and I started doing the same thing again. One thing I knew for sure was that I wasn't going out that window again—because there was no window. The hole in the wall I'd made the day before had been patched with a solid piece of plywood."

Stead was more determined than ever not to quit. "So I ran and ran, and just like the day before I saw those white spots. Directly outside the barracks a bunch of guys were working out with weights. I ran right through that plywood patch and cleaned out that group."

Stead never passed out again and eventually, "I got to the point where I could hang with the best of them. Day by day I was losing weight and gaining strength." But he had been on Parris Island for three months; the platoon he'd entered training with was about to graduate while he hadn't even started actual training. In his mind, he'd failed.

"I was crushed. I just gave up. I told the DI, 'Sir, I don't care what you do to me. I'm giving up, I've had it. You guys have beat me.' He realized I was serious, and instead of coming down on me he took me into his office, and we had a long talk. He promised to get me into training in one week if I agreed to hang in there. He kept his word. I finished basic training, and then went through infantry training, and by the time I got to go home I had been there eight months." Eight months in boot camp may be a world record, but Stead's trip home was even more astonishing, and it underscored how time and military training change young people into adults in a wide variety of ways.

Stead reported, "I weighed 185 pounds when I got home—with muscles. I got off the Trailways bus and walked down the street to the school where my mother ran the cafeteria. She was behind the cash register when I walked in. I said, 'Hey, lady, how about some chow?'

"She looked at me as if I was the rudest person she had ever met and went back to counting change. Then I said, 'Mom, it's me.' My mother didn't recognize me, my own mother."

In eight months, the U.S. Marine Corps had changed him from a fat adolescent into a rock solid man. "No longer was I going to be called jelly belly, fat boy, blubber bumper, and all those wonderful things they call you when you're an overweight teenager. I could look at myself in the mirror and say, 'My God, man, you're normal!'"

Clearly, basic training involves a balance between food and exercise, discipline and satisfaction. Some young people are eating machines, so even with all the food available, at night there were recruits who craved something extra to eat. Sometimes, as one member of Val Nicholas's platoon did, they take action. "There was a vehicle called the Roach Coach that came around at night selling to the sergeants things like candy bars and other stuff we weren't supposed to eat. We had this one guy who was so stealthy, he would sneak out a window, crawl around the building, crawl under cars and around them, until he reached the wagon. He would buy a bunch of snack food and repeat his process in reverse: under and around cars, staying in the shadows, crawling in the dirt to avoid detection, until he got back to the barracks—where he would then sell it to us for ten dollars a candy bar."

The formidable "Snake Pit" is an honored tradition at Lackland Air Force Base. The Snake Pit is a strategically located table where TIs sit and eat during chow. As trainees go through the chow line the TIs selectively pick out people to answer questions about their military knowledge or to be inspected. Nobody wants to be summoned into the Snake Pit, but basically it's unavoidable. A female was called over because "the TI said I was treating the food line like a model's runway, meaning my hips were moving when I walked." The best example of the inevitability of a visit to the Snake Pit is the experience of a trainee who reported that he was ordered there because the TI said that the trainee looked like he was "intentionally trying to do everything right, so that he wouldn't be ordered to the Snake Pit."

TI Tim Price happened to be there for one of the most memorable days in Snake Pit history. Price recalls the day. "Some TI had a dink throw himself out of the chow hall for an infraction. He had the dink place one hand on his own shirt collar and his other hand on the seat of his trousers. When he was in position he started to throw himself out of the chow hall door, but he missed and ran into the center beam just as the major was walking in. He split his pith helmet open and knocked himself on his can. The major, without a word, turned on his heel and left the chow hall."

The Upper Hand:
Military Courtesy

"The origin of the hand salute is uncertain. Some historians believe it began in late Roman times when assassinations were common. A citizen who wanted to see a public official had to approach with his right hand raised to show he did not hold a weapon. Knights in armor raised visors with the right hand when meeting a comrade. This practice . . . in early American history sometimes involved removing the hat. By 1820 the motion was modified to touching the hat, which has since become the hand salute taught today."

—*The Soldier's Blue Book*

THOSE PEOPLE WHO HAVE served in the military share a common tradition and even, it can be said, a common language that is not readily understood by Americans who didn't serve. A part of a common language is greeting each other, and in the military that is summarized by the hand salute that is rendered between officers and enlisted troops. Civilians greet each other, of course, but they do so in a variety of ways. All military people do so the same way, and in some respects it is uniquely satisfying because it has a beginning and an end, and it is unambiguous.

In fact, one of the first things a recruit learns is how to properly salute an officer. Paul Setmaer (air force, Lackland, 1977) remembers how he learned that lesson. "We got our uniform the second day, but they didn't have name tags on them, so everybody was called a 'pickle,' we were just nameless people in green uniforms walking around. After we had our lunch we came out of the mess hall and walking around the corner came this person with a silver bar on his collar. We hadn't received any instruction what an officer even looked like yet. So as I passed him I said casually, 'Hey, how you doing?' In retrospect that was a mistake. I was immediately pounced upon. That 1st lieutenant taught me how to salute correctly and explained that I had to salute every officer. I knew how to identify a 1st lieutenant but I had no idea what other officers looked like. So for the rest of that day I walked around saluting every person I passed. Playing the saluting game was fun; every officer corrected me and every other recruit ignored me."

"Saluting may be the easiest thing you learn in basic," according to Michael Nichols (Marines, San Diego, 1995), who eventually served three years as a Drill Instructor. "But there are people who have difficulty learning it. While working as a DI I saw the widest variety of salutes imaginable. I had people saluting with their left hands, their palms facing away from their eyes. I had people miss their cover and touch their foreheads, even almost poking themselves in their eyes. I even had people give the Hitler salute. All of this gave DIs an opportunity to get to know these people a lot better. Much, much better."

The army was no different. "There are a lot of details to a simple salute," explains Michael Volkin (army, Ft. Leonard Wood, 2001). "Everything matters, from the angle of your feet to the way you raise your hand. We had people saluting everywhere on their face from their chin to their hairline. We did have people who poked themselves in their eye—or their glasses."

While most people assume knowing when to salute is obvious, there are nuances. For example, when should a recruit salute a car? The answer: When an officer is in an official vehicle, which can be identified by special license plates or flags.

Recruits are taught that the salute is properly executed with the right hand to the tip of whatever cover, or hat, is being worn. In the salute the fingers and thumb are extended and held together, with the palm facing down. The outer edge of the hand is canted slightly downward. The navy salute is slightly different, as the palm faces down and is rotated an additional 90 degrees in toward the shoulder. Supposedly this dates back to the days of sailing ships, when sailors worked with tar and pitch so their hands were always filthy and tilting the salute inward would hide that.

David Fisher (army, Ft. Leonard Wood, 1969) was on detached duty when trainees were taught when, where, and how to salute, so he missed that instruction. A few nights later, he remembers, "I was marching back and forth guarding an abandoned field when the lieutenant drove up in the jeep to check on me. I knew I was supposed to salute him, but I had a rifle on my shoulder and I didn't know how. So I made it up. I took the rifle off my shoulder and put it in front of me in a parade position, holding it with my left hand, then put the palm of my right hand against it—about mid-chest—and saluted. The officer just looked at me dumfounded, then finally said, 'Where'd you get that one, Flash Gordon?'

"And suddenly I realized that was exactly right! That was exactly the way Flash had saluted."

Mike Volkin (army, Ft. Leonard Wood, 2001) had a battle buddy who put his own twist on the salute. "He had his own style of doing everything, and his attitude was that his way was the right way and the way everybody else in the world was doing it was the wrong way. Rather than snapping a sharp salute, he made it into an elaborate circle. He'd sweep his arm way out wide, as if his hand was coming in for a landing. The Drill Sergeants did not like that, and so they created a special smoking for him. The next day, for twenty-four straight hours, he had to change into a different uniform every hour and report to the Drill Sergeant's office to salute him properly. He would be in a PT uniform with boots on and change into his battledress uniform. The next hour he'd have a different cap on, the next hour his Class A uniform. Every hour for twenty-four hours he had to put on a different combination of pants and shirt or equipment, report, and execute a proper salute."

After Johnny got through basic training, he
Was a soldier through and through, when he was done
Its effects were so well rooted,
That the next day he saluted
A Good Humor man, an usher, and a nun.

—lyrics from "It Makes a Fellow Proud
to Be a Soldier" by Tom Lehrer

The Recruit's Body of Work: Physical Training

W HILE THERE IS ABSOLUTELY nothing similar to basic training, there are ways for the prospective trainee to prepare for it. There are things a young man or woman who has enlisted can do before reporting that will make the experience more palatable. Rod Powers, who reports on the military for *About.com* and is the author of several military guide books, writes, "I'm often asked for the best method of getting in shape for military basic training. For those who have spent their teenage years in front of the TV, here is a little secret for building arm and shoulder muscles: Begin by standing outside . . . with a five-pound potato sack in each hand, extend your arms straight out to your sides, and hold them there as long as you can. After a few weeks move up to ten-pound potato sacks, then fifty-pound potato sacks, and finally get to where you can lift a one hundred-pound potato sack in each hand and hold your arms straight for more than a full minute.

"Next, start putting a few potatoes in the sacks, but be careful not to overdo it."

Once again we are put through the five events of the Physical Combat Proficiency Test. We crawl and squirm through the low crawl as if we were sneaking up under enemy machine guns. We run around hurdles and leap over a pit, cutting, and shifting, spinning and twisting, as if a torn-up battlefield stood between us and our objective . . . We hang by our arms, hand-over-hand, way down the rows of horizontal ladder . . . simulating either a rope-bridge crossing or a game of tag with Tarzan. We run through the 150-yard man carry, staggering up a gradient with a soldier on our backs, saving perhaps a wounded buddy from capture. And finally, without even a minute to catch our breaths, we are clustered on the track and begin the mile run. In the bleaching sun, slowed by sweat-soaked fatigues and heavy leather boots, we thunder around the track. . . .

We have all suffered through four weeks of painful physical training. It tore our muscles at first, broke them down before it would build them up. But now we begin to see the results. Virtually all of our scores have improved impressively.

—Peter Tauber, *The Sunshine Soldiers*, 1971

Physical conditioning has always been the core objective of basic training, the goal being to turn out soldiers, sailors, Marines, and airmen in top physical shape and able to fulfill their missions. You can't run through enemy fire if you can't run. If you're in bad physical condition, carrying a sixty-five-pound rucksack, a weapon, ammunition, and other equipment becomes an unendurable chore. When you are in poor shape, everything is a trial, and you become not only a burden but a danger to your comrades. How to achieve the objective of well-conditioned troops has been a matter of fierce debate for a long time, and it is safe to say that there has been no resolution of it.

Conditioning programs have varied greatly. In 1943, Tony Vaccaro (army, Centerville, Mississippi) remembers, "The obstacle course consisted of a lot of ropes and wooden barriers. It was climb something, go down something, run between rubber tires, and crawl through the mud. Whatever you did, it was in the mud.

"One exercise was a little strange, though. We actually exercised our index finger. As they explained, we were training our index fingers to pull the trigger. It wasn't that hard: Pull the trigger, stretch out your finger, pull the trigger, stretch out your finger. We were told to stretch our index finger in and out three hundred times a day. I was standing next to a guy who must have weighed three hundred pounds, and believe it or not he was sweating from this exercise because his hand was so heavy it was hard for him to hold out his hands."

Through the years the physical requirements for military service have continued to evolve, sometimes because of genuine advances in the understanding of how to become physically fit, but occasionally for absolutely no logical reason. As a group, American youth are in relatively poor physical shape, and converting them into tough warriors requires a considerable investment in time, effort, and commitment.

Generally the army requires a minimum of one hour of PT daily, but in an environment in which there is insufficient time to mold all troops into fighting condition, much of physical training is a compromise. In 1981, for example, according to Anthony Shaffer, "The army had just adopted the new PT tests, which consisted of push-ups, sit-ups, and the two-mile run. The run was the biggest deal. They were still making us run in boots and fatigue pants, their reasoning being that if you were going to fight wearing fatigues and combat boots, you should train in them. The result was that everybody got shin splints. We had people constantly going on sick call and missing training because they were forcing us to train in combat boots." Fortunately, that changed a long time ago and today recruits wear running shoes while training. In combat, though, soldiers still wear boots.

At the beginning of training, very few troops are prepared for the intensity of the workouts. "You're in so much pain all the time that you keep thinking, 'How can I get out of this?'" Thomas Kilbride (Marines, Parris Island, 1980) recalls, "It was probably two months into it before you really got into it."

Like most trainees, James Crittenden (army, Ft. Sill, 1992) forced himself to push through the pain. "The hardest part for me was the running. I could run a short distance because I'd played football, but when it came to running two miles, that was really hard for me. I managed it by telling myself to keep going, just keep going. I thought about the millions of people who had gotten through this, and I figured if all of them could do it, then I could do it. And then after a while it got fairly easy, and when I graduated I was able to do it." And those people struggling to get through it now can think that if trainees like James Crittenden could get through it . . .

In 2010 the army completely revised its basic training conditioning program, ostensibly to make it more relevant to contemporary warfare. The program reduced the reliance on the traditional exercises like sit-ups, jumping jacks, and push-ups. "In the past we've only done push-ups, sit-ups, and a two-mile run," said General Mark Hertling, then commander of army training. "Frankly, none of those address the kinds of things soldiers are asked to do in combat. No one is being asked to run five miles in combat, but they are being asked to zigzag across streets. So we do have more focus on sprinting rather than long distance runs. We are being asked to train people who grew up in an environment where the focus was more on playing with their thumbs than playing with a bat. How do you train them to hump a rucksack at nine thousand feet in the Hindu Kush? We're building tactical athletes."

The most common phrase any trainee will hear is "Drop and give me twenty"; twenty push-ups. "We did endless push-ups, just endless," recalls Paul Steingruby III (army, Ft. Jackson, 1987). "They said that by the time we left we'd pushed the ground down two inches. We had one guy who was the biggest screw-up in the company. So he spent probably three-quarters of basic doing push-ups. And he got better and better at them. We had a command sergeant-major who prided himself that he could do more push-ups than any of the trainees. At times he would get down next to trainees just to show then that he could outdo them. It was the ideal set-up.

"Well, this guy had gotten into great shape. One day he got caught playing grab ass and the Drill Sergeant gave him fifty push-ups to do. The sergeant major, true to his nature, got right down next to him and started matching him push-up for push-up. They both breezed past sixty, then seventy, when the recruit got through eighty the sergeant major started to lose steam. But that private just kept doing his push-ups effortlessly. The sergeant major eventually got up and recovered and without a word walked out of the area. He never challenged anyone again."

While Steingruby III did not explain what punishment the recruit received for embarrassing the sergeant major, probably it wasn't more push-ups.

Many young people enlist in the military service because they want to improve themselves physically, as well as develop discipline. Discipline they certainly got, but they also got something else the real world rewards: competition. Steingruby said, "The idea was that if you finished in the top two in any physical test you didn't have to do KP, so it got pretty competitive. We had two official PT tests for grading, one after we came in and another before we were able to graduate. The five events at that time that we were tested on were the horizontal ladder, push-ups, sit-ups, run-dodge-jump, and the two mile run."

For Nadine Gabrielle-Miran at Ft. Leonard Wood in 1996, a combination of excessive punishment and the focus on PT turned her into a physical fitness star. "There was a certain door in the barracks we were not allowed to use. One night they dismissed us, which meant we were allowed to get to the pay phone to call home. I was one of the fastest runners in the platoon, and I raced out the approved door and got to the phone first, but some of the other girls told the Drill Sergeants I'd cheated by using the closed door."

She explained to the sergeants that she was merely fast, and then, realizing what would happen if they didn't believe her, began pleading with them. She failed to convince the cadre that she was telling the truth. "As punishment, for a week before graduation they made me get up every two hours, put on my full battle dress, meaning thirty to fifty pounds of gear, and report to the nighttime security desk. Most of the time I couldn't get back to sleep, and so I would read or write letters home, but I also began using that time to work on my push-ups and sit-ups. As a result I got better and better at PT, and when we were tested I ended up getting the PT award."

The Marines, of course, take great pride in having the most grueling physical training. Fifty-nine of the total 1518 hours of training are devoted solely to PT. Dan Bierbaro (Marines, Quantico, 1966), who was a platoon commander during a leader training program, remembers those long challenging runs. "This was during the summer, and it was brutally hot. There was a series of hills that you had to run up and down, and a lot of guys passed out. In fact, they'd had some fatalities on the hill trail, people literally had died of heat exhaustion. So they put an ambulance on the top that had a tub of ice in the back. If a guy passed out they'd grab him and literally throw him in that tub of ice to bring down his body temperature."

"You had to pass the Marine Corps Physical Readiness Test or you got sent back to do two more weeks of boot camp," explains Richard Hubbard (Marines, San Diego, 1969). "You had to accumulate 325 points out of a possible 500. I had played athletics in high school, but by the end of boot camp I was in the best shape of my life. I remember thinking, the Marine Corps has successfully turned me into the physical specimen I absolutely never wanted to be!"

While the requirements for female trainees are different than for males, they are no less grueling. As Heather Borden (navy, Great Lakes, 2002) explains, "Our instructors had a phrase that they used called 'making it rain.' Indoors. When somebody screwed up they would close all the windows in the barracks, shove all the racks against the walls, and force us to work out until literally condensation dropped from the ceiling.'"

"We called it 'The Circle of Death,'" explains Philip Landon (navy, Great Lakes, 2005). "They would run us in a circle until everybody's sweat had pooled on the deck and converged in the middle of a circle. We considered it some sort of satanist ritual, except the blood was replaced with sweat. One day while we were doing it, a recruit grabbed his heart and fell over. We didn't know what to do. We thought he might be dead. Another recruit ran over and started doing chest compressions. They brought in a gurney, and several guys carried him out. And as I watched it happen I realized that two other guys just walked out. They took advantage of the situation. They were dressed in their PT gear and what we found out later was that they went directly to the Pizza Hut and were gone for nine hours."

"We had to do a lot of running at Lackland," Cindy McNally remembers, "but they were pretty good about it. One thing they made us do was run with our hands across our chests to hold our breasts, because in 1975 they felt if we didn't run with our hands in a cross across our chests we might loosen something."

By 2000 the requirements had changed for women in the Air Force. Tracy Harrell was in a mixed flight, in which men and women trained together. "During regular PT sessions we ran the same amount, did the same amount of push-ups and sit-ups and calisthenics as the men. For the PT test, though, we didn't have to do as many sit-ups and push-ups and we got a little more time for our runs."

But just to make training a little tougher, when Kihm Winship was at Lackland in 1968, "During PT we weren't even allowed to spit. Sometimes, after calisthenics and running, we were tempted. But those who spat into the grass were ordered to find their spit, pick it up—and eat it." No further comment required here, except, perhaps, from the Centers for Disease Control and the National Institutes of Health.

Each service establishes its own physical fitness standards required to graduate from basic training or boot camp. In some respects—principally the time allotted and the number of repetitions required—these standards are very different, but not for any easily discernible reason. For example, in addition to other events, the Marines require trainees to do crunches and pull-ups, while the other services do not. There are also different standards for men and women. In the air force, for example, men must complete a 1.5-mile run in less than about 12 minutes, but women have nearly 14.5 minutes to cover the same distance. In the Marines, males are required to do pull-ups while women do flex arm swings—which means hanging from a bar. A lot of the differences in requirements for men and women have to do with tradition, with women generally considered the weaker sex, but that certainly is less true than ever before. As results of marathon races have proven, for example, many women can run longer and faster than many men.

Which proves that it is no longer entirely accurate to guarantee that every recruit who completes basic training or boot camp will leave as a new man. Now a substantial number of trainees will leave as new women.

Men and Women for All Seasons: The Weather Factor

I T IS GENERALLY AGREED in the military that there is a best season to go through basic training—and, of course, that is any
time except the time you've done it. In basic, there are only two
types of weather—too hot or too cold. The United States is in a
temperate zone, an ironic misnomer, since temperate zones are
characterized by weather extremes. It's the extremes that veterans
remember with the greatest clarity. Robert Oxford was at Great
Lakes in December 1965 through January 1966, "The coldest place
I have ever been in my life. It was 8 degrees, there was always
snow on the ground, and a wind was blowing off the Great Lakes.
We put on as much clothing as permitted, but I always thought
part of our training was learning how to deal with the cold. Our
chief petty officer's strategy for keeping warm was 'keep the line
tight, keep it tight. Get close to the guy in front of you. Don't stop
till your dipstick goes into the oil well in front of you.'"

There is snow on the ground for most of the winter at Great
Lakes, and as the Drill Instructors of Parris Island protect their
sand fleas, the CPOs at Great Lakes value their snow. The navy
takes great care to make sure its snow is guarded by trainees. As

instructors warn recruits, "That snow belongs to the United States Navy, and your job is to make sure nobody takes it."

In 1967 Tom Fitzsimmons remembers, "It got down to –20 degrees, and they would get you up at 3:00 A.M. to stand guard outside over the Dumpsters. One thing that was absolutely guaranteed—no one was going to steal those Dumpsters. Not that they didn't want Dumpsters, it was too cold!"

Philip Landon was there in the winter of 2005–2006. "The first day I got there all I saw were people in trench coats and ski masks. I thought that was pretty strange—until we went outside. Then I couldn't wait to put on my ski mask. We would dress in a skull cap covered by a ski mask, a sweater, trench coat, and a white scarf. We wore black leather gloves over white cotton gloves and we wore two pair of socks. And we were supposed to train in all that. It was like we were too big to actually move. In the navy the barracks are called ships, and we lived in a brand new ship. Everything worked very well in our ship, with one exception—the heat. When we went to sleep at night it was 30 degrees in the building. The heat worked on a sensor, and in order to get it to kick on you'd have to walk in front of it. We'd spend all night trying to get the heat on so we could go to sleep for a few minutes."

At Great Lakes in 2009, the appropriately named Jacob Blizzard remembers, "It was so cold I was freezing through my ski mask. My breath was condensing on my eyelashes; ice was literally forming on my eyelashes, and my eyeballs were freezing shut. It was awful. Our CPO told me that it was a great way of building character. Right, I thought, especially if that character is a snowman."

It also got cold in the South, as Curtis Baskin learned at Camp Sibert, Alabama, in 1943. "Going south for the winter from Pennsylvania I just froze my butt off. We were living in tar paper shacks with just two pot-bellied stoves, one on each end of the building.

One platoon, I remember, really wanted to ace the morning inspection, so they poured water all over their floor to mop up—and it turned to ice."

Tom Jones was on bivouac at Ft. Gordon on a freezing cold night in October 1962. "The first night we camped in the woods the temperature went down to about 8 degrees. It was cold and damp, and it just cut right through your bones. We were all freezing, and we didn't have the proper equipment for it. Early in the morning the first sergeant told me to go line up the troops. I tried to get everybody up and out, but they weren't interested. Their response basically ranged from, 'Fuck you,' to the much more polite, 'Go screw yourself.' Nobody wanted to move. When I reported that to the first sergeant he got furious. He started kicking down tents, and truthfully they weren't much better to him than they had been to me. He finally threatened one recruit, 'I'm warning you, you keep up this shit and I'll make sure your ass goes back to jail.'

"From inside the tent I heard this voice reply, 'Well, goddam, at least it's warm in jail.'"

When Homer Hickham was at Ft. Leonard Wood in the winter of 1966, he learned that "If you left your fatigues out at night, in the morning you practically had to break them to get into them. I used to take my fatigues to bed with me to keep them warm."

There is a real debate over whether it is better to go through basic when it's too hot or too cold. Eric Dell (navy, Orlando, 1994) admits "I graduated from high school in June and I had a choice when to ship out. I decided to go to Orlando, Florida, in the middle of August. August in Orlando, Florida? I hadn't even started boot camp, and already I'd made my first mistake. The very idea of Orlando in August is now appalling to me, and I wonder what was going on in my mind when I picked that date. Apparently, not enough."

All the services have instituted procedures for dealing with training in extreme cold or heat, and at one temperature or another, training is directed to become less intense and demanding. Usually, above 90 degrees, all physical activity that isn't essential is halted. This, of course, is ironic considering that for a decade we have been fighting in Southwest Asia, where temperatures are routinely substantially higher than that. Hydrating—learning when and how much water to drink—has become an important aspect of training. Tynesha Brown (army, Ft. Jackson, 2010) reports, "We had a lot of heat casualties in South Carolina because people weren't drinking enough water. Our Drill Sergeant warned us, 'It gets hot here and you ain't drinking enough water, eventually you're going to pass out. Unfortunately, if you do, it's going to take some time for the medics to get to you, so I might have to cool you down by peeing on you.' You should have seen people going for their canteens."

Matt Farwell says that Ft. Benning in 2005 was ideal training for desert warfare. "It got to Heat Category Five, which is 95 degrees, pretty regularly. They would tell us that the Georgia heat and the desert heat were equally bad. There was a strong emphasis on knowing proper hydration techniques, and people would get on me because I would drink twelve or thirteen canteens a day. I'd also steal salt packs from the mess hall because it helps replenish electrolytes. We had to have a parachute cord attached to our lapels the whole time, and after every canteen we drank we would have to put a knot in the cord. The Drill Sergeant could tell just by looking at that cord if the private was properly hydrated. That was a big part of our training because, as they emphasized, our bodies were our weapons."

Replenishing electrolytes is important, of course, but the services could not make up their minds about whether or not trainees should take salt. For many years, salt tablets were issued, and trainees were instructed to take them regularly. Then, somebody asserted that taking salt merely made you thirstier and was counterproductive to remaining hydrated. More recently, it has become popular to take salt in the form of expensive commercial hydrating drinks, but it's really plain water—available almost everywhere—that makes the difference, and too little or too much of it is not good.

"The heat was dangerous," remembers Robert Hanna, who was at Ft. Benning at the same time as Farwell. "Dealing with it was an ongoing challenge. We did have somebody in another company die while several others got sick from either not being hydrated or being over-hydrated."

While instructors have a litany of tales that they tell recruits to shape behavior, as Mike Zaleuka saw at Ft. Benning in the summer of 2009 sometimes the worst stories are true. "We were running hundred-yard sprints that had to be completed in seventeen seconds or less. One of the guys in my platoon started walking funny, then he passed out . . . They called for the ice sheets, which are literally frozen bed sheets to be used on him and took his temperature.

"His real temperature was 107 degrees . . . He topped out at 108 degrees. He went into cardiac arrest, but they brought him back." Two days later Zaleuka wrote to his parents, "Our battle buddy, and brother, passed away this morning due to complications from his condition. It really sucks around here right now, everyone is down and some people are really torn up over the situation."

Heather Borden (navy, Great Lakes, 2002) will never forget the "challenging" result of learning how to deal with the heat. "The navy wants you to stay good and hydrated by drinking all this water, but they do not give you many opportunities to release said water after it has run its course. You can't just raise your hand and be excused to go to the bathroom. There are set times to use the bathroom."

A dutiful navy recruit, Borden had already drunk a large portion of the eight canteens of water mandated daily by the time she reached her first classroom lesson. She was dying to get to the bathroom.

"But nothing is that simple. Taking our seats was a big production. All eighty of us had to be in perfect unison, as judged by a megalomaniacal RDC running that hour's lesson. We were all lined up in descending height order, standing next to our desks. First he called out in an ultra-authoritative voice, 'Take.' Then we did it again, and again, until the RDC finally was satisfied with the first half of the command. After mastering 'Take,' we got ready for 'Seats.' Everyone had to sit in unison, which was in the eye of the leader—and his eyes apparently did not work in unison.

"Bathroom breaks are not given until we have mastered 'Take' and the far more complicated 'Seats.'

"On a day when my bladder was about to explode, this was torture. The longer the 'Take. Seats.' charade continues, the closer I got to losing control, losing it right down the inside of my leg. Up and down. Up and down. Suddenly, for a brief moment I lost my 'bladder control' concentration—and felt a warm drop of fluid running down my inner thigh. Normally, that would have been enough to make me regain my composure and 'tighten up.' Normally, but I was in boot camp and there was nothing normal about spending twenty minutes learning how to sit down.

"The sensation of that initial trickle was heavenly. I had never felt anything so divine. Finally, I just gave it up. 'Screw it,' I thought and just let it all flow. So while everyone else was busy concentrating on the art of sitting down, I was enjoying the immense relief from peeing my pants. I didn't think about the consequences; I did not care."

Of course, a large pool was forming around her feet, and because the floors were not level, pretty soon the unfortunate girl in front of her noticed the trickle. "There was nothing I could do,"

Borden lamented. "My act was about to be revealed, which would have an impact on everything that happened from then on in boot camp, and perhaps even my navy career. My life was about to change forever because of those eight canteens of water. And then the girl in front of me said the most beautiful words I have ever heard, 'I think you spilled your canteen.'

"'What? Oh, yeah. Silly me. Spilling my canteen of *water* on the ground. I'm such a klutz.'

"The megalomaniacal instructor excused me to get some paper towels to clean up the *water* that I had accidently dropped from my canteen. When I returned the girl in front of me even volunteered to help me sop up the mess. I accepted, naturally."

The Mess Hall Actually Should Be Called the Neat Hall: KP

There's dirty work to be done in the army, And it's not much fun
It's the kind of work that's done, without the aid of a gun
The boys who work with the cooks in the kitchen, Holler out for
   peace
For they have to do the dirty work, And they're called the Kitchen
   Police.
   —lyrics from "Kitchen Police (Poor Little Me)," Irving Berlin

I N THIS SCENE FROM the 1932 movie *Pack Up Your Troubles*, Laurel and Hardy are on KP during World War I basic training. They are loading garbage pails filled with food scraps on a hand-pulled wagon:

OLIVER HARDY: If you'd done as the sergeant told you we wouldn't have to be doing this.
STAN LAUREL: Well, I knew what to do.
OLIVER HARDY: Well, why didn't you do it?
STAN LAUREL: I just couldn't think of it.
CHEF (angry): Hey, hurry up and get back here with those cans.

OLIVER HARDY (To Chef) : Say, what do we do with this stuff?

CHEF (sarcastic): You trying to kid somebody? What do you suppose you do with it? Take it to the general.

STAN LAUREL (To Hardy): What do you suppose the general wants with this?

OLIVER HARDY: There you go asking questions again. Why don't you try doing as you're told once? Don't you know that you've got to follow the curriculum of the army, with discipline. Com'on. If the general wants it, he can have it.

No one survives basic training without the details—these particular details being unpleasant assignments ranging from working in the kitchen to guard duty. Throughout military history KP, standing for kitchen police, kitchen patrol, or perhaps the more accurate, keep peeling, has become the best known. While private contractors run mess halls today, the memories survive. In the past getting through basic without serving KP was almost impossible, because a certain number of workers were needed in the mess hall every day. As Peter Tauber (army, Ft. Bliss, 1969) wrote in *Sunshine Soldiers*, it couldn't be avoided:

" 'Tauber,' whispers the Drill Sergeant during closed-ranked inspection, 'You're going to KP tonight, and do you know why?'

" 'Yes, Drill Sergeant,' I reply.

" 'Why,' he asks, testing me.

" 'I don't know, Drill Sergeant,' I answer.

" 'Why did you answer *yes*, then?'

" 'Because you're not supposed to answer *no*, Drill Sergeant,' I reply truthfully.

" 'You lied when you said you knew why, didn't you?'

" 'Yes, Drill Sergeant.'

" 'You're going to KP for lying.'

" 'Thank you, Drill Sergeant.'

" 'For what?'

" 'For telling me why, Drill Sergeant.' "

KP means working in the mess hall, doing any task from food preparation to cleaning. In general, KP was considered the worst detail. Some basic veterans will argue that guard duty on a frozen night is worse, but KP had its own unique and memorable charm. Trainees who have cleaned a grease trap on a warm day are still searching for an appropriate metaphor to convey the horror of it.

At Lackland, Kihm Winship recalls, "It was predictably awful. I remember the briefing at 'Hell's Kitchen.' A sergeant told us that the wash water was 170 degrees and would take the flesh off our hands and arms if we didn't wear the gloves. We wore the gloves. He didn't tell us that the Amazon Pine Oil would take the polish off our boots, though, and it did. The heat from the pans and wash water swelled our hands. The garbage cans full of slop (marked 'edible' and sold to pig farmers) pulled our ligaments loose from their moorings as we hauled them away."

In military service, there are lessons to be learned from every task, no matter how banal, lifelong lessons that survive all subsequent experience. Winship continued, "We began work at 3:00 A.M. and were ordered to leave all our personal possessions behind, including wedding rings," said Winship. "Some newlyweds balked at this, and our sergeant told us, 'If you take it off she won't die. If that worked, I'd have done it years ago.' "

A military unit feeds hundreds of people every meal, a formidable enterprise, and no task is too small or too unimportant. For example, when Saul Wolfe served KP at Ft. Dix in 1958 his Drill Sergeant demanded that every single thing on every table in the mess hall be perfectly aligned. "We thought we had it right, but he was so crazy that he made us stand on either side of the dining room and stretch a string between us—to make sure that all the salt and pepper shakers were lined up in a row."

Preparing food in an institutional environment does not require a pot. It requires *lots* of pots. Tidying up is not a matter of wiping a few surfaces but instead requires a thorough hosing and swabbing and hosing again. One morning at Ft. Dix in 1963, Herb Cohn was put on bacon detail. "It wasn't complicated. It consisted of taking this huge slab of sliced bacon and laying it out on dozens and dozens of sheets to be cooked. It was awful. By ten o'clock in the morning I was completely covered with this white greasy slime. For the next couple of weeks, no matter what I tried, I couldn't get it washed away. There wasn't any known soap that could get rid of that stuff, and it had this horrible smell. After that I didn't want to eat a slice of bacon for at least two years."

As Jerry Leitner (army, Ft. Sill, 1944) points out, "When you get KP there are better jobs than others. The worst job was cleaning out the grease trap. It was a big metal box that collected all the grease and cleaning it out was the single ugliest and most repulsive job you could do. The best job of all was peeling potatoes."

Peeling potatoes was clean, perhaps, but it also was the most tedious job. Peeling potatoes meant peeling hundreds and hundreds and hundreds of potatoes. "There must have been a thousand pounds of potatoes, and there were three of us assigned to peel them," remembers Marty King (army, Ft. Leonard Wood, 1969). "Fortunately there was a big potato peeler, a large tumbler that knocked the skin off them. This is when I really began to understand the military. The potatoes were stored in a cold room and we began dragging the bags across the floor toward the peeler. The E-6 in charge asked us, 'Where y'all think you're going with them things?'

"I told him, 'We're gonna put them in the potato peeler.'

"He looked at me like I was the crazy one. 'You can't use that peeler,' he said. 'You'll get it all dirty.' Then he handed us each a knife that was about four inches long, including the handle, and suggested we better get right to work.

Unfortunately for Harold Fritz (army, Ft. Knox, 1966) peeling potatoes was only the beginning of his worst day in basic. "They brought in this huge mound of potatoes, and it was just awesome. I said to the guy I was working with that we were going to be there all night. The mess sergeant said they had a potato peeler, but it wasn't working. I figured I could fix it. I did, sort of: When we put in full-sized potatoes they came out about the size of golf balls.

"We reduced this huge pile down to several bushel baskets, but when the mess sergeant saw what was happening to his potatoes he wasn't happy. So he assigned me to what was basically permanent KP. But then I saw an opportunity to get on his good side. In the old mess hall they had a little bathroom. In that bathroom they had an officer's section, a non-commissioned officer's section, and a section for trainees. The floor tile in the officer's section was in bad shape and had to be redone. The mess sergeant asked me, 'You know anything about doing tile?'"

Fritz knew absolutely nothing about tile, other than you walked on it and it stayed down. "'Yeah, I can lay that tile,' I told the sergeant. I figured this was my chance to get on his good side. How hard could it be? You put down some glue and pushed the tiles into it. The problem was that when I laid the tile we had to spread this black gooey stuff on the floor, but I didn't know how much of it to use. So I put down whatever we had, which turned out to be too much. When I laid the tile on top of it and patted it down, this black goo started spurting out between the seams. I scraped it all away and when I was done it looked pretty good. I figured it would dry and be okay."

He figured wrong, of course. "The next the morning the officers came in for breakfast and one of them needed to use the bathroom. I was feeling pretty good about it right up until I heard the crash. A few seconds later this officer came out of the bathroom with this black gooey stuff stuck all over his hands and his uniform. Maybe in a different situation I would have laughed, but this was *this* situation. He was fuming. There was nothing I could do but stand there, realizing that my life as I had known it was about to be finished.

"I found out that when he went into the bathroom his boots hit a loose tile, which flew out from under him. He went flying, and as he did he kicked up more tiles, exposing all of this black glue, which ended up on his hands and once-immaculate uniform."

Fritz had KP for the next few days in a row, and at one point, the mess sergeant, who apparently had developed some bizarre appreciation for the magnitude of Fritz's mistake, said "I understand you have some leadership potential, but you sure stepped in some manure this time."

"Maybe," mused Fritz, "but it wasn't me who did that stepping."

The Pain Is in the Details: Guard Duty

PROBABLY THE SECOND MOST common detail is night guard duty, although no trainee has ever been assigned to guard anything that might actually need guarding. Guard duty usually consists of standing or marching near some installation or item of equipment that is either unlikely to get stolen or is already impregnable. Popular among the former is an abandoned wooden building that served as barracks during some war long ago. Guard duty is really only for training purposes. By himself, or even with a few other new troops, the trainee would be incapable of repelling an attack. Even if an intruder identified himself as, "the enemy," there's very little a trainee could do to stop him. "You had your rifle and they gave you one cartridge," explains Dan Blatt (army, Ft. Dix, 1962), "but you weren't allowed to actually put it in your rifle. I guess they felt it was too dangerous to give a trainee a loaded weapon."

Guard duty is usually performed in one-hour increments, but few things in life move as slowly as one hour on guard duty. As hard as a guard tries, usually the only thing he or she can think about for the entire hour is how long one hour can last. Sometimes, though, as John Langeler learned at Great Lakes, it can be extended—and extended. "The punishment we got for some infraction was to stand guard over a Dumpster for four hours in the freezing cold in the middle of the night. We were literally guarding garbage to prevent someone from stealing it. To make sure we knew what we were doing, at some point during your tour an officer would sneak up on you. In response you had to say, 'Halt. Who goes there,' and make sure whoever it was knew the password. One night the password was 'Peter Pan.' The captain approached and the guard from my platoon challenged him, 'Halt! Who goes there?'

"The captain replied with the correct password, 'Peter Pan.'

"Unfortunately, the kid had forgotten the password. So instead of permitting him to pass," Langeler reported, "he said sarcastically, 'Okay, Peter Pan, fly yourself over here and show yourself.'

"Which is how he ended up standing watch every night for the next two weeks."

In the barracks at Lackland, explains Kahlil Ashanti (air force, Lackland, 1992), "We had dorm guards. There was a large metal door with a small window, and each night one of us would be responsible for standing at attention behind that door all night, refusing admission to anyone who did not have the proper ID and knew the password. The TIs definitely would test us. When ordered to show their identification, they would show anything: Dunkin' Donut coupons, porn, a package of condoms, anything to make us laugh. Then they would try the nice guy, 'Okay, good job, let me in. I got some work to do.' After that, if the guard refused to open the door they would threaten him, 'Let me in this damn dorm or I'll rip off your balls.' Sometimes the guard would then open the door—and immediately get smoked for falling for that trick and opening the door. The ultimate penalty was being recycled, which meant you went back several weeks in training." The lesson is that, when you're dealing with the enemy, trust no one, and learning to harbor a healthy skepticism is an excellent preparation for adult life.

A lot of details are just make-work; there is a reason details are called "details." Generally, they are time-consuming, labor-intensive, banal, often useless, and at times confusing: The one question a trainee never, ever, is allowed to ask under any circumstances is simply, Why?

For example, it can be argued that there is no rock in the world that actually needs to be painted, but that doesn't stop the military. Richard Hubbard (Marines, San Diego, 1969), "Our DI needed to take some time off. So the whole platoon had what was called KP maintenance. They took us over to the navy base, which was right next door, and assigned us to chores. My job was painting rocks. All the rocks around headquarters buildings? My job was to paint them."

"We painted everything at Lackland," says Cindy McNally. "We painted trash cans, we painted steps, and we painted rocks. If it wasn't moving, we painted it." Unlike other tasks assigned during basic training, learning how to paint rocks actually will have some application later in military careers—as the painted rocks in places as disparate as Kansas and Afghanistan, Vietnam and Djibouti prove.

"We also cut the grass, and then we cut it again," said McNally. "The grass was always being cut whether it needed it or not. That was a terrible detail because San Antonio in August is very hot and humid, and we'd be out there in fatigues, steel-tipped toe covers to protect your feet, and a cover. We were never allowed to be without a hat. We'd be pushing a manual lawnmower cutting acres of grass that had been cut yesterday and the day before and was going to be cut the next day."

Troy Bayse (army, Ft. Benning, 2010) may have seen the most unusual detail in basic. "I don't know what this guy did, I never found out, but every day he was out in front of the company area sorting rocks. There was just this big hole, and they had him taking out rocks and sorting them into two piles, big rocks and small rocks. Whenever we weren't training he would be in that hole. There was nothing brutal about it, just putting the big rocks over here and the little rocks over there."

Part of the challenge of those details was figuring out creative ways of getting out of them. It is well known that basic training affords young people few opportunities to exercise their creativity—with the sole exception of finding ways to avoid details. At Lackland in 1968 David Taylor was given clippers and told to trim the hedges. "I started to clip a circular hedge around a banana tree. As I was doing that I noticed there was a gap between the tree and the hedge, so I pushed through the hedge and began trimming it from the inside. From the inside where no one could see me. When I was sure no one was looking I sat down, hidden completely by the hedge. This worked very well—until another airman started clipping the hedge and noticed there was a gap between the hedge and the tree. He noticed it because he saw me sitting there. I signaled him to be quiet and waved him inside. He sat down with me and the coast was clear. For obvious reasons we couldn't talk, but we definitely bonded. When we heard a sergeant shouting to everyone else on detail to finish up we slowly stood up and began clipping the hedge." Another detail performed to perfection.

Michael Mamett (army, Ft. Leonard Wood, 1960) relied on the one method guaranteed to avoid all details. "My method was simple: I just paid someone ten bucks to do my guard duty for me. We also had to pass a test with an M-1 rifle, which I could never do, and so I had to pay someone else to do that for me, too." Clearly, Mammet exhibited those characteristics essential for success in what would eventually become the business of outsourcing.

Of all the punishment details, PT remains the most memorable. Tom Seaver got caught with dirt in his rifle while at San Diego and had to do an exercise known as "Up and on shoulders. First I had to hold out my rifle, which weighed eleven pounds, straight in front of me. Then I lifted it over my head, then I held it out in front of me again. Up and over again and again. I had to do it over and over—not until *I* was exhausted, but until my Drill Instructor was tired. And then when he got tired, another instructor replaced him. It went on for more than three hours. I thought my arms were going to fall off—but I guarantee you from that point on I had the cleanest rifle on the entire base."

Shawn Herbella made the mistake of reporting for morning PT without his T-shirt neatly tucked into his trousers. Only in military logic would a uniform called "fatigues," which are meant to be worn for filthy, sloppy, sweaty work, have to be neat, clean, and often starched. "I knew it was a serious mistake as soon as I saw the senior Drill Instructor looking at me. He told me to get in a front leaning rest position, the push-up position, with my feet on a two-foot high pile of sandbags in front of the entire formation.

"I had to stay in that position for the entire formation, during which he gave this long speech. I fell and hit my face a couple of times. I think he forgot I was there, or maybe that's what he wanted me to think. At the beginning of training the front rest position was punishment, but towards the end it became laughable. I can't begin to figure how many times I was in that front rest position, but eventually I could do it all day long. My arms and chest got so built up it was easy. And it was an effective way of making us focus on the small things."

Dennis Stead's most memorable lesson came when his platoon failed a barracks inspection. "His point was that we were screwing up and he told us we were garbage. And as garbage we belonged in the Dumpster. So he opened up the door and made us get in. It was big enough to hold maybe twenty human beings, so when you get sixty people in there it gets pretty hot and uncomfortable. Fortunately for me I was one of the last to get in because the guys at the bottom really caught hell. The people on the top did the best we could to help them get air, but it was tough. They didn't keep us in there too long because somebody really could have got hurt. Sometimes you think these DIs were sick in the head, but they definitely knew how to make their point."

First Class Instruction:
Classroom Work

O F THE WEEKS OF training Dr. Sam Rollason (army, Ft. Jackson, 1972) survived, one day still stands out. "One of the series of classes that will probably remain embedded in my memory as long as I live is the venereal disease classes. I am sure that the army spent a great deal of time and money in developing what went into the making of those films. Psychological studies have probably been done on their effectiveness in combating VD. The psychology that was used was simply this: to gross out as many men as possible, thereby scaring them into a short-lived state of celibacy while in basic training. But from personal observation the scare tactics last only until a good-looking girl passed by.

"Then came the big moment of the films. They were crammed full of rotten cocks, some half-eaten away by VD. There were lovely close-ups . . . of yellow fetid discharges from the vagina of a girl whose labia minora were seemingly eaten away, putrid looking peckers running pus from the urethra.

"And then we marched to lunch."

As actor-comedian Kahlil Ashanti states, "They always warned us to make sure if we were with a woman to wear a 'jimmy hat' or 'body bag,' which was slang for a condom, but once they showed me those films they didn't have to worry about me ever again. Those films scared me out of ever touching a woman as long as I lived."

A considerable amount of time during initial training is spent sitting in classrooms learning the basic structure of the military service and essential tools for survival in the military. All recruits are taught the Uniform Code of Military Justice, including regulations governing race relations and sexual harassment, alcohol and drug awareness and treatment, career progression, and even some antiterrorist training. Each service also instructs trainees on its history, structure, customs, and courtesies. The air force, for example, allots more than forty hours to educating airmen about various aspects of life in that branch, as well as financial management, human relations, lifestyle, and fitness. Every minute of instruction has been planned in detail. As TI Tim Price explained, "TIs had lesson plans they had to follow. Lesson plans were divided into two parts: Required Instruction and personalization. It was always recommended that personalization be kept to a minimum . . . Every lesson had a format: Introduction, Application, Motivation, Instruction, Performance, and Feedback."

Marines are taught essentially the same material, including the proper use of equipment and how to make a rack, but they also receive hands-on instruction in swimming. Army trainees receive instruction in each of the seven Core Army Values: loyalty, duty, respect, selfless service, honor, integrity, and personal courage—which happen to spell out the mnemonic LDRSHIP, as well as the rules and regulations governing daily life in the military.

At boot camp navy trainees study a wide range of topics from the proper way to iron a uniform to firefighting and damage control aboard ship. Boots also learn how to tie a variety of traditional knots and, naturally, swimming.

To graduate from navy and Marine boot camp you have to pass a swimming test. "You had to stand on a line nude for half an hour while they talked to us," says Robert Oxford (navy, Great Lakes, 1965–66). "We jumped from a high diving board feet first into the pool. I can remember the sting to this day. You had to do a couple of laps back and forth, that's all it was."

John Langeler explains, "The kids who didn't know how to swim struggled a lot. If you couldn't swim, they would kick you back to the next company to start all over again. They taught us how to jump in the water, remove our trousers, tie knots in the bottom of the legs, then kick up in the air and pull them down really fast, and they would actually inflate for a while. Then you would put them under your arms and they would support you. When they deflated you would do it again."

Brian Deever (Marines, Parris Island, 1993) admits, "I didn't know what swimming entailed. When they told us to jump into the water in uniform and a weighted back pack I thought, that doesn't seem like a great idea. That thing isn't going to float. They taught us how to put everything in garbage bags and pack it tight inside your backpack. I didn't know how to swim but I jumped in with my backpack on and my only thought was, I'm going straight down. But it floats! It floats! If you pack it right, it floats."

The training is actually quite demanding, even for enlistees who knew how to swim before they entered the service. But there are genuine nonswimmers among the enlistees.

It was because of swimming that Canaan Brumley (navy, Great Lakes, 1992) went through boot camp twice, once in the navy as a trainee and a second time in 2005 with a Marine platoon, as a documentarian making the film *Ears, Open. Eyeballs, Click.* "In the Navy to qualify you had to jump into a heated pool off a high diving board, about twenty-five feet, tread water for five minutes, and then swim one lap around the pool. If you couldn't pass the test you had to take remedial swimming classes until you qualified."

Before he joined the navy, Brumley was an excellent swimmer, "but you don't realize how long five minutes is until you try to tread water that long. After five minutes my arms and legs felt like Jell-O and I was out of breath. I was struggling. It was about then that some of the other people decided that they wanted to race around the pool as fast as possible and started kicking other people in the face. Just as I was getting started I got kicked in the throat. I immediately lost my breath and went to the bottom of the pool. I was drowning. I couldn't breathe, I could barely see. I have very bad vision, without correction I'm just about legally blind, and in the water I wasn't wearing my glasses. I could vaguely make out some navy guys at the bottom of the pool with breathing apparatus so they could rescue anyone struggling. I was struggling. I could see their eyes through their masks, but I couldn't tell if they were trying to give me any kind of directions because I couldn't see well enough. I reached out to one of them for help, but he pushed me away. I guess that's because they want to keep people from panicking and ripping off their breathing gear. Instead I got jabbed in the side by a long pole, and I grabbed hold of that pole and they pulled me out of the pool. I think the divers are there only if you black out and can't save yourself.

"I had to go back and take the test again on another day. There are people who think that lives aren't in jeopardy, but unfortunately, as I learned when I was making the documentary, that isn't true."

Making decisions about how to train is difficult. Leaders must decide the fine balance between realism and danger, between potential injury in realistic training and skill in the ferocious reality of armed combat. The danger is real, and sometimes the outcome is tragic. "The Marines have to go through a far more difficult process, which involves going into the water in full uniform and swimming a lap with a backpack. When I was filming my boot camp documentary, there was a bad case of Strep A, a respiratory disease, going around. When you put a large group of people in one big room, work them hard and only give them a few hours' sleep, their immune systems are going to be compromised, germs are going to spread, and everybody's going to get sick. When you're in boot camp the last thing you do is admit you're sick because you're afraid it's going to get you held back so you won't graduate with your unit. You don't want to stay in boot camp one minute longer than you have to, so you'll do anything possible to avoid that.

"A really bad Strep A had spread through the whole unit when I was filming. This one kid apparently was very sick when he got in the pool for the endurance test, but he didn't tell his Drill Instructor. He went under the water and swallowed some water and the combination of the water and Strep A was too much. When they pulled him out of the pool it was obvious he was in very bad shape. He was turning white. The DIs were so hard-core they were still screaming at him, telling him to get up on his feet and be a Marine, shouting in his ear that Marines don't die until they are told to die.

"But this trainee never regained consciousness. I don't think he survived more than a couple of minutes after they pulled him out of the pool. It wasn't anybody's fault, but there was nothing anybody could do to save him."

The subject matter of classroom instruction has changed considerably through the decades, but in the past these classes were often pitched to the lowest possible level. For example, during the Cold War trainees watched an instructional film entitled *How You Spot A Communist*. Among the tips, look for people hanging out near the base, who may have an accent and ask a lot of questions.

From the documentary *Basic Training* by Fred Wiseman:

"This time, gentlemen, we're going to be brushing the front teeth, then we'll be brushing back and forth in this manner right here. We'll be brushing back and forth on the front teeth. Put the tooth brush in your mouth. Brush. Good, short, fast strokes, back and forth."

According to Philip Landon (navy, Great Lakes, 2005), "Coming out of boot camp the only thing you really are expected to know" is how to be what is called an undesignated sailor. Basically, the rate is known as bosun's mate. You learn the basics, how to moor up a ship, tie knots, and paint. That's all you are expected to know."

Apparently the most difficult part of classroom instruction is staying awake. You would think that something as exciting as a military subject would keep students transfixed, but that is not the case. It is one thing to load a high-powered military rifle with live ammunition and then get to actually shoot it or fight with pugil sticks, but it is far more difficult to sit through hours of droning, interminable classroom instruction that precedes the live firing. Generations of men and women in uniform have been subjected to sessions that serve less as training than mental torture. For example, exactly how long does it take to teach a recruit how to properly brush *all* their teeth. Ron Weisberg (army, Ft. Knox, 1969) remembers "vividly that we had to sit through a movie presentation about the proper way to brush your teeth. We had kids from parts of the country who had to be taught these things."

As Anthony Shaffer (army, Ft. Gordon, 1981) explains, "The classes were pretty lame. They were taught at about an eighth-grade level, and we would have to sit there for hours. It was pretty boring because they wanted to make sure everybody got the point, and so it just went on and on. It was after PT, after eating, and people would be there nodding off. We'd watch heads go down and suddenly jerk up. Up and down. Up and down."

Wyatt Draggoo (air force, Lackland, 1993) succumbed and fell fast asleep. "I was startled from my slumber by the TI shouting, 'DRAGGOO! What the hell do you think you're doing?'

"I leaped out of my chair to attention, and as my brain was warning me, don't do this, my mouth said, 'I'm checking my eyelids for holes, Sir!'" As a result, Draggoo spent an extra week in basic, eventually becoming a performer in air force shows.

Trainees are tested on the information taught in these classes and have to pass them to graduate, but these courses are all geared to make sure that everyone can pass them. If a trainee fails, he receives remedial training and is retested. The objective, after all, is to produce troops who can do what they are supposed to do. The military is not testing their ability to learn generally, their study habits, or their capability to remain awake during stultifying instruction. And no final exam will ever rival the test Sam Ehrman took at Camp Grant in 1943. "We had been taught how to dig a slit trench. It was a two-man job and it had to be deep enough and narrow enough for a tank to drive over it. When it was done, we got down inside, and they drove a tank right over it. Then the tank stopped and whirled around two or three times. The sides started crumbling, but when the tank drove away and you were still alive—that's how you knew you passed the test."

Finding Yourself in the Military: Learning Navigation

SGT. TOWER: Now I'm gonna tell you gen'lmen how you find you way when you lost. You better listen up. What you do, you find the North Star and the North Star show you true north accurate all year round. You look for the Big Dipper and there are two stars at the end a that place in the stars that look like the bowl on the dipper, and they called the pointer. They them two stars at where the water would come out the dipper if it had some water, and out from them on a straight line you gonna see this big damn star and that the North Star and it show you north and once you know that, Gen'lmen, you can figure the rest. You ain't lost no more.
                    —an excerpt from *The Basic Training of Pavlo Hummel*,
                    a play by David Rabe

THERE ARE MANY IMPORTANT skills a trainee must master, and most of them require frequent practice to gain and maintain proficiency. The ability to navigate in unfamiliar terrain, to get from one place you don't know, to another place you don't know—that's the province of lower animals and a very small number of gifted humans. There is instinct in land navigation without a GPS, and it requires a sense that most humans don't possess. Teaching land navigation ultimately involves taking trainees to a point in the middle of the woods, and then having them use a map and a compass to find another point, an exercise that often results in frustration for both the trainee and the cadre.

Of course, some instructors have the brilliance to reduce complicated techniques to a simple solution. At Camp Shannon, Texas, in 1944 Milton Pike was taking a class in navigation, trying to locate an enemy position. "Our instructor told us that finding the enemy was probably the easiest thing we would learn. He said, 'The best way to find the enemy is to go out and let them shoot at you.' When someone is shooting at you, you know you've found the enemy."

Norman Batansky was on a logistics trial at Ft. Jackson in 1969, during which "We had to get from point A to point B, which were probably around three or four miles from each other, carrying a full backpack, rifle, and other equipment. We were put in different teams of two men. My partner and I started walking toward point B and all of a sudden we saw a road. Hey, let's follow the road. We followed it for a while and eventually we found a bar and grill. So the two of us, with all our gear including our rifles, went into the bar and asked if anyone knew how we could find this point B. We showed them the map and one person knew exactly where it was. 'Can you drive us there?' So we got into his car and he drove us close to the point. We gave him a five-dollar tip. It turned out we were the first team back, and because of that we were given the next day off."

This is not in the spirit of the exercise, of course, but most important is that Batansky and his buddy might have overpaid, since five dollars was a great deal of money in those days, and it was well known around Fort Jackson that the local populace was happy to perform this service for free.

Following Orders

"I wonder if you have any idea what this means to a former second lieutenant of horse cavalry. It's wonderful to be here with you at Parris Island. You'll notice we brought some rain with us . . . It was fascinating to see your obstacle course and the 'slide for life.' It reminded me of trying to get a bill through Congress. We don't have an alligator or sand fleas, but we got some people in Washington who could double for them in a pinch.

"But since this is the Marine Corps and it was supposed to be real hot here, I planned to keep my remarks short—no more than an hour or so . . . One time I addressed a group of Marines. I told them a favorite joke of mine and was disappointed when they didn't laugh. And I thought maybe I'd gotten the delivery wrong or they didn't quite understand it or something. And then the commanding officer leaned over to me and whispered that they were standing at attention, 'They're not permitted to laugh.' So, just to play it safe: At ease, and feel free to laugh. That's an order."

—President Ronald Reagan addressing Marine
trainees at Parris Island, June 4, 1986

The Worst of It All:
The Gas Chamber

The Training of the Soldier: Defense Against Chemical Warfare. Under the direction of the Chief of Chemical Warfare Service, Signal Corps, the recruits are issued gas masks and given training in their care and use. Trainees watch a film showing "Bringing in the men gassed in the attack on May 2, 1918 to evacuation hospital #2." Twenty percent of all casualties were gas; 70,752 men were casualties during World War I. Most of them recovered.

—WWI training film

THE GAS CHAMBER IS one of the oldest—and without any doubt the least popular—elements of basic training. It was introduced during World War I to prepare troops for the chemical warfare they would encounter on Europe's battlefields. At that time trainees were taught to put on a gas mask within six seconds from the instant a warning was given. Cavalry troops also had to learn to put the mask on their horses as well. To teach trainees how to function while wearing their masks for long periods, as on the battlefield, they had to perform various other activities while wearing them. One film from those days shows a baseball game in progress, with all of the players wearing their gas masks. It also appears that random "gas attacks" were part of the training, in which harmless smoke canisters were dropped without any warning, and troops had to respond. In some respects, this is very similar to the training currently being given in basic to increase awareness of the use of IEDs in Iraq and Afghanistan.

The horrific effects of deadly gas during the First World War led to its banning by international convention afterward, but it hasn't stopped some leaders from using it anyway. Incapacitating substances, like tear gas, are still used in some situations. In training, all branches use CS gas, o-chlorobenzylidene malononitrile, a nonlethal substance used commonly by police for riot control. Trainees have to go inside the gas chamber, remove their mask, and perform a simple task, usually just answering a question. Generally the entire experience inside the gas chamber lasts only about a minute, just long enough for a trainee to experience the effects of the gas, although for many trainees that will seem like the longest one minute of their lives.

MASTER CHIEF: In this fifth week of training, you all will be tested in the proper way to use your gas masks. Below decks on a ship at sea this mask may well save your dumb-ass lives. The drill is simple. Step one—put on the mask. Step two—turn on the air supply. Step three—who can tell me what step three would be? Zimmerman raises his hand. Yes, Recruit Bagel?

ZIMMERMAN: Breathe.

MASTER CHIEF: God damn, Bagel, if you could get in shape I'd put you up for nuclear engineer. That's right, you all, breathe. The way the drill works is like this. You enter the chamber with masks on. A tablet of tear gas is put on a hot plate. On my command you will then take off your gas masks. Do not do it before I give the command. Then one by one, left to right, you will say your name, where you are from, and then your social security number. When everyone in your row has done this simple thing correctly you may exit the tank. Should you get sick during this process it better not be on my shoes. Is that understood?

ZIMMERMAN: I'm not sure about my social security number.

—from the play *Basic Training* by Daniel Landon

At Ft. Jackson there is a sign just outside the entrance to the gas chamber which reads, "Are we having fun yet?"

Almost every trainee goes into the gas chamber with a plan for beating—or at least reducing—the effects of the gas, plans which range from keeping both eyes tightly closed to simply not breathing. All these sophisticated techniques have the same outcome: They don't work at all. Trainees are kept inside the chamber just long enough to insure that, as is inevitable, everybody inhales. "I thought I'd be able to handle it," Robert Hanna said, "but once that mask came off I felt like I couldn't breathe. There was just snot and spit everywhere. They made us stay in that room for about a minute. I never expected it to be as bad as it turned out. Although not necessarily a fastidious person, I found the snot and spit nearly as unpleasant as the effects of the gas."

"It was the worst thing I have ever done," Troy Bayse says flatly. "The absolute worst. That is the only time in my life I literally thought I was going to die. You walk into this room in groups of ten or more. It's hot as heck in this room, and it feels like the pits of hell. In the middle of the room there is a pan on a burner and they drop the chemical in there and the fumes begin spreading all through the room. Before you even take off your mask the gas gets all over your skin and it burns, like someone holding a match to your skin. Then you pull your mask away from your face for just a few seconds. You feel it a little bit, and then you put your mask back on and clear it. The point of that is so you understand that the equipment works; it does what it is supposed to do. Then you know you can trust it."

You know you must remain calm . . . but, naturally it is not as simple as that. Reality never is. Once the trainee removes the mask, his eyes spew tears the volume of Niagara Falls—it *is* called "tear gas," after all—and he begins to choke on the CS vapor. Donning and clearing a mask is not all that difficult in dry training, and, indeed, most troops can get very proficient at it. Trying to do it while hacking like someone suffering from the end stages of a terrible disease may be a bit more difficult. The equation is irrefutable: The more hacking, the less successful in clearing the mask quickly, which results in still more hacking.

Bayse remembers clearly how the cadre insured that every trainee got the full opportunity to enjoy the CS experience. "What they made us do was put our rifles between our knees, hold our helmets in one hand, take the gas masks off, and put the helmets on properly, including buckling it, then hold our rifles up in the air in one hand and our gas masks up in the air with your other hand. It isn't so easy. As soon as you take the mask off, those gases rush into your nose and throat and lungs, your skin is on fire, your face is on fire. You can't breathe because those gases are filling your lungs, you're coughing and snot is flying everywhere. Your heart is palpitating. You're not going to die, but you feel like it. There was one person who passed out, but they dragged him out of there real quick.

"I just remember putting my helmet on and knowing I was done with it, but you can't leave until everybody in your group is done. And the guy in front of me was having trouble. First he dropped his mask. Then he couldn't buckle his helmet. He was so bad that I started beating him on the back, screaming at him to hurry up, 'I can't breathe.' The harder I hit him the worse he got. You couldn't *pay* me to do it again."

Mitchell Friedman (army, Ft. Leonard Wood, 1969) has never forgotten his visit to the gas chamber. "I was a little older than most of the other people in my platoon. I'd already graduated from law school, and so the Drill Sergeants felt a little freer to kid with me. In fact, they often used me as the demonstrator for different instruction. When somebody had to get thrown in hand-to-hand combat, it was me. When they wanted to demonstrate the proper way to hit someone with a pugil stick, it was me. They knew I could take it. So the day we went to the gas chamber I wasn't surprised when our Drill Sergeant told me, 'You're gonna like this, you're gonna be the first one in and the first one out. You're gonna show everybody what it's like.'

"That sounded okay, get it over with. 'Good,' I said. 'Where's my protective mask?'

"'That's the thing, see: you're the demonstrator. You're going in without the mask. Your job is to show everybody what happens if they don't wear their masks.' Well, there was a seriously bad idea. If the object was to scare everybody else, I definitely succeeded. I walked through as fast as I could, which was still not nearly fast enough. I came out of there with liquid coming out of every orifice, coughing, choking, fighting to get my breath. I guarantee that from that point on everybody else paid close attention to the instructions."

"Watching people come out of the gas chamber is one of the funniest things you will ever see . . ." claims Drill Sergeant Kevin Robert Meade, ". . . until you have to go in. The only one who enjoys it is the guy outside taking pictures for the cycle book. Even as an instructor your skin is going to burn a little. But generally, it isn't dangerous. Once, though, I had a person who broke the seal on his protective mask and took a breath, then tried to reseal it. It didn't work, he threw up inside his protective mask. At that point he was going to choke to death because there was no place for the fluids to go, so we had to rush him outside and rip off his mask."

Each service has its version of the gas chamber, and the requirements vary slightly. "The anticipation was almost as bad as the experience," Brian Deever remembers. "The Marine Corps gave us training ahead of time in how to use the gas mask. They told us what to expect, and then they marched us down for the practical application. There was a shack in the middle of the woods, and they took about ten people at a time inside. While you're waiting to go in you could see people on the other side coming out. It wasn't pretty. You could see the mucus coming out of their noses, you could hear them coughing and desperately trying to breathe, and you begin thinking, this can't be good. This is not what I want to do right now. I began wondering, now what have I gotten myself into?"

When Deever and his fellow boots entered the gas chamber, they had to remove their masks and hold them in their right hands, so the instructors could see clearly that they were off.

"And then we had to recite the alphabet, just so you can get the stuff in your lungs to know what it feels like. At that time it was the worst thing I'd ever done in my life. I don't remember ever realizing exactly how long the alphabet was until that moment."

Thomas Burke (2004) explains how it was done at Ft. Benning. "We had to go in with our masks on and recite the soldiers' creed, 'I am an American soldier. I am a Warrior and a member of a team. I will always place the mission first,' and it goes on. But then we'd break the seal on the mask and recite it again. It was a lot tougher the second time. When we finished they'd send us out the door to do the walk of shame, with everybody coughing, drooling, snot dripping out of our noses."

Rather than a gas chamber, the navy refers to it as the "confidence chamber" and strongly advises trainees to "eat light" that day. In addition to the gas chamber, navy training includes firefighting experience under tough simulated shipboard smoky conditions.

In some cases, the traditional training in the skills of coughing and choking amid a cloud of riot control gas has been replaced by the much more comprehensive NBC training—Nuclear, Biological, and Chemical training—which introduces trainees to the other, perhaps greater, battlefield dangers that exist. As Kahlil Ashanti remembers, "When we began chemical warfare training I thought they're going to teach us how to avoid chemical weapons. But the first thing they did was show us how to use atropine to fight the effects of nerve agents. Apparently atropine is an antidote to certain nerve agents. They gave us an atropine needle, which was about the length of family-sized toothpaste tube, and told us that when we were exposed to a nerve agent we were supposed to take this long needle and simply inject it into our heart.

"Simply inject this long needle directly into our heart? There is nothing simple about injecting a long needle into your own heart. When our instructor explained that to us, I started looking around and it was obvious everybody had the same response I did: What is this guy, fucking nuts? Who's gonna do that?

"Then they told us we were going to practice doing it. Excuse me? Practice it? What they did was give us a retractable needle, like a children's toy, to practice with."

In addition to the gas mask in NBC drills trainees have to put on full-body protective gear that provides head-to-toe protection. Ashanti continued, "Then we were taught how to put on MOPP-4 (Military Orientated Protective Posture) full body coverage, essentially Hazmat suits, within a prescribed period of time, then you had to clear your gas mask, so it didn't fog up. The training lasted a couple of days. We had a certain amount of time to put on the suit, the boots, the mask, then tape around our ankles and wrists. Once in the suit we had to look around and drink from a tube to prove we could function. To pass the test all we had to do was keep breathing. If you couldn't breathe, you failed." Because these suits are impervious to anything from the environment, they trap body heat and hold it. Every bit of the heat. On a hot summer day in the desert, almost anything is more bearable that being in an airtight MOPP-4 suit.

There were immediate, more mundane fears associated with this kind of training. Ashanti recalls that, inevitably, there were some people in the unit who practiced poor hygiene. "So we would sit in the classroom as the TI told us about nerve agents that would peel away our skin or turn our insides into gelatin, so they would flow out, but meanwhile all we could think about was I hope that guy with bad hygiene didn't use this mask yesterday. We were more worried about touching the spittle from that guy's mouth than our organs turning to liquids."

In the end, however, the mere prospect or theory of something is not nearly as instructive as being actually exposed to it, and there is nobody who ever forgets the experience in the CS chamber, especially when the instructors sought to lengthen and thus intensify the lesson by having the recruits unmask and then perform vocally, as Deever did in reciting the alphabet. Occasionally trainees had to recite their social security numbers or the General Orders, or they had to sing a song. It was typically diabolical that the instructors often chose the Marine Hymn or the Star-Spangled Banner or some other music designed to be sufficiently long to insure choking and gagging and the rest of it. Neither the Marine Hymn nor the National Anthem will ever be sung as quickly as they are sung in a gas chamber, and with the encouragement of CS gas, the entire score from the opera *The Marriage of Figaro* can probably be sung in under a minute.

At least Tracy Harrell got a break. When she went through training at Lackland in 2000 the air force was converting its gas chamber into an NBC chamber, "So instead of having to go through the whole process we had to get into our full chemical gear, do all the face mask fittings, practice putting it on and taking it off—and then they waved an ammonia-type substance in our face. You had to tell them if you could smell it or not. If you couldn't smell it, that meant your gear was on correctly. If you could smell it, you had to do it again, but if you couldn't you were done. It was not a hard decision to make. We did the chemical warfare training on the honor system."

Turn Your Head and Cough: Health and Fitness in the Military

"What's all the excitement?"

"A hornet!"

"Where?"

"On Sarge's nose."

"Suppose it'll sting him?"

"Shh! There'll be a lot of disappointed people if it doesn't."

—from the comic strip *Beetle Bailey* by Mort Walker

COLLEGE STUDENT BEETLE BAILEY joined the comics page army in March 1951, and he apparently spent the next several *years* in basic training at Camp Swampy. Beetle, along with continuing characters Sgt. Snorkel, Lt. Fuzz, and Miss Buxley, eventually moved into an extraordinarily dysfunctional infantry unit, but it appears that he spent more time as a basic trainee than anyone in history.

There is nothing which gains an officer the love of his soldiers more than his care of them under the distress of sickness; it is then he has the power of exerting his humanity in providing them every comfortable necessary and making their situation as agreeable as possible.

—Baron von Steuben's *Revolutionary War Drill Manual*

Among those things guaranteed to occur during basic or boot camp is that some percentage of the recruits will get injured or become sick. This is not surprising when you consider that a large number of young people, from disparate parts of the country, are thrown into a highly stressful situation, often under difficult conditions, during which they have to radically change all of their habits. The majority of recruits will be physically challenged in basic training more intensely than ever before in their lives. These stresses all combine to magnify the medical risks that most people encounter in their normal lives.

Without question the worst medical disaster to strike basic training facilities was the Great Flu Epidemic that swept the world in 1918 and resulted in more than twenty million deaths. As Edward Coffman wrote in his book *The War to End All Wars: The American Military Experience in World War I,* "On November 5, 1918 General March cabled General Pershing about the situation: 'Influenza not only stopped all draft calls in October but practically stopped all training.' . . . Recruits, particularly those from rural areas were the most vulnerable, as over 60 percent of the men in the army who had the disease had been in uniform less than four months."

Feeling their way through the catastrophe, commanders quarantined the camps. They tried to reduce crowding without success and consequently just ordered the windows in the barracks to be kept down. To reduce transmission of the virus, troops were instructed to hang sheets between beds and between the tables in the mess hall. Men not living in barracks furled the sides of their tents and put out their bedding to air every day. If a man still contracted the disease, about all the doctors could do was put him to bed, give him aspirin, try to keep him warm, and hope he would not get pneumonia.

There have been other outbreaks of disease in basic training camps, some with the unintended consequences feared by all leaders when they have to make decisions under less than optimal conditions. In 1963 for example, four recruits died and 12,000 recruits at the Naval Training Center, San Diego, were placed in quarantine after an outbreak of meningitis. Three years later, recalls TI Mike Harrell, "Lackland was shut down completely because of another big meningitis scare. But this was in the middle of Vietnam, and so they had to continue to train troops. They opened Amarillo Air Force Base as a training center and staffed it with Lackland Instructors. When we got there an officer put out the word, 'You're here for one purpose: to train troops. I don't care how you do it. I don't want any beatings, but this isn't Lackland, and you train the way you want to train. We looked at each other and said, 'Oh boy!' For the next six months we got away with things we wouldn't have even thought about doing at Lackland."

"When one of our boys came down with meningitis," remembers Homer Hickam (army, Ft. Leonard Wood, 1966), "it put our DIs in an absolute panic. As they told us, 'Meningitis is a killer,' and warned us that if it spread we might be put in quarantine. To deal with it we were taught how to make 'sneeze sheets.' Essentially they were barriers between bunks. They issued us metal rods that fit on the end of the bed and used it as a mast. Then you pulled up your shelter half, draped it over the stick to make kind of a little sail-shape, then tucked it under your mattress, so if you sneezed you wouldn't be sneezing on anybody."

By 1968 at Ft. Jackson, Richard Goldman explains, the sneeze shields were slightly different. "You had to prop it up so it was kitty-corner on your bunk so it created a triangle. That way if you sneezed it would go not into the center of the barracks, but instead it would just nestle in your own equipment." Of course, this strategy made little sense when you considered that the trainees spent all their other time squashed together—in the field, in latrines, in the mess hall—coughing all over each other with no sneeze sheets to protect them.

Ken Dusick was put in quarantine at Ft. Ord in 1969 when cases of meningitis began turning up. "We wore a white tag on our chest to indicate we were in quarantine and we weren't permitted to leave the section of the base in which we were training. If they caught you outside supposedly you'd be court-martialed, but they didn't really enforce it.

"They took every precaution in that situation to keep us away from anyone who was infected. We had Christmas leave and as I was getting ready to go home I ate some bad food and got so sick I was actually delusional. When I stumbled into the camp hospital I was hyperventilating. The first thing they did was strap oxygen over my mouth and nose. Hyperventilating means you're getting too much oxygen, so they decided to give me more oxygen—which was potentially deadly. They couldn't understand why my heart rate, blood pressure, my pulse, everything was rising rapidly. Some doctor looked at my fingernail, which had turned blue. He realized what was happening and ripped off the mask, maybe saving my life.

"They put me in a room in the hospital. Gradually my stomach got better, but when I woke up the next morning the man in the bed right next to me had died from meningitis. So much for the quarantine."

While infectious diseases are always a concern, most illnesses turn out to be minor and don't interfere with training. It's the physical injuries that cause the most annoying problems. "We had to do the ladder bars every day," explains Mitchell Friedman. "I wasn't an athlete, and so when I heard something pop in my shoulder and felt a sharp pain I went right to the infirmary. The diagnosis was 'Not a significant shoulder separation.' Not a *significant* shoulder separation? What does that mean? To me it was like being 'slightly pregnant.'" Slightly pregnant or not, Friedman returned to finish basic training.

Most trainees have not made a habit of falling out of bed at 5:30 every morning, doing calisthenics, and then running two miles before breakfast. The result of unusual or sustained physical activity is often injury, and injuries are common in basic training, even among those with a long history of being compulsively fit.

One of the trainees in basic with Anthony Bayse at Ft. Dix in 1989 "was Mr. Muscles. He was 180 pounds of pure muscle, perfectly cut, definitely a high school football player. He had a big mouth, but nobody messed with him because he was a threatening presence. Everybody was afraid of him. I, on the other hand, was a walking shadow, 6' tall and a thin 160 pounds. For some reason when we were learning pugil stick fighting, which supposedly taught bayonet or rifle fighting, our Drill Sergeant decided that I should go up against him. A pugil stick is a pole with padding on both ends, and you use it to block your opponent and then hit him. Somehow I don't think he took me seriously, and during this fight I managed to break his finger hitting him. Or he broke his finger hitting me. It didn't matter. That finger was still broken." While not a life-threatening injury, to Mr. Muscles this was worse—death by embarrassment. *Sic semper tyrannis.*

For many people, a broken finger may seem disfiguring, painful, and damned inconvenient, but for others, like Chicago White Sox left fielder Carlos May, it had the danger of destroying a career. When sportswriter Bill Madden (army, Ft. Jackson, 1969) entered basic, he was already aware that May's career almost ended when he blew off the tip of his thumb while learning how to fire a mortar in Marine Corps training. And the potential loss of his own finger dominated Madden's consciousness. He said, "The whole time I was in basic I kept thinking, don't shoot off your finger, don't shoot off your finger. I wasn't ever within miles of a mortar, but it was constantly, irrationally on my mind at the firing range, during exercise, anything physical we did. Maybe I wasn't going to play in the major leagues, but I was determined to leave basic training with both of my thumbs and all of my finger tips!"

At the start of the training day, recruits who feel ill, have somehow injured themselves during the previous evening, or are simply looking for an excuse to avoid training present themselves for sick call. Those who miss training for more than a couple of days risk being recycled, which means assigned to another platoon and forced to repeat the previous few weeks. So rather than complain, they endure—although at times it becomes absolutely necessary to see a medic. Saul Wolfe (army, Ft. Dix, 1958) had an officer who was possessed of a monomaniacal desire to set every conceivable record for training recruits. "We worked harder and longer than any other unit," said Wolfe. "As a result the one record he achieved was putting more people in the hospital than anybody else. We actually had guys who were too sick to get to the hospital. This officer thought it looked bad that so many people were going on sick call. So in order to go to the hospital you had to pack up everything you owned into your footlocker and carry that footlocker down to the supply sergeant and turn it in. If you were too weak to do that, then you couldn't go on sick call."

Generally, the most common complaints are blisters, rashes, poison ivy, and easily spread fungal conditions like athlete's foot and even ringworm. It seems like there is always someone in training who has some type of contagious, itchy thing that lasts for days or weeks and, as explained in those documentaries that showed on a map the inexorable spread of communism across Eastern Europe, can't be stopped—and can't be scratched, either. Or at least shouldn't be scratched, because the brief, ironic, blessed relief that results from digging nails painfully into the raw skin is followed by increased contagion and more unbearable itching. Anthony Shaffer claims he was "attacked" by ringworm while on bivouac at Ft. Gordon in 1981. "It started off on the inside of my left arm and ended up covering two-thirds of my body. I watched it spreading, and there was nothing I could do to stop it. It was like this itch that gradually attacked my entire body. The hardest thing was not scratching it. I tried to be a good troop, but eventually I went on sick call. They didn't know exactly what it was, some kind of fungus, so they gave me an astringent for it. That just made the fungus angry. I went back three times before they figured out what it was. They finally gave me a pill, which took another week to work."

When people are ill, rest is often deemed to be the most effective cure, and occasionally a significant percentage of a training unit will be in the barracks, resting. Even resting in the barracks, just relaxing while others are sweating in the field, has consequences that are deleterious to health. Air force TI Mike Harrell had a trainee who went on sick call complaining of a minor ailment and was given two days bed rest in the barracks. "It was some type of upper respiratory infection, nothing serious, but those things can get worse and become dangerous. The only thing he was supposed to get out of bed for was chow. These two days were over a weekend, but I decided to go in and check on my flight. As I walked in the dorm I saw this recruit—and he had a full cast on his leg. I couldn't figure out why they were treating URI with a leg cast. 'What the hell happened to you?' I asked.

" 'I broke my leg, Sir.'

"Okay. 'Can you tell me please how you managed to break your leg while on bed rest?'

" 'Well that was just it, Sir. When I was getting out of bed to go to chow I slipped on my blanket and broke my leg.' " This should have been fair warning that this man was not to be trusted with a loaded weapon or hand grenades, and that he needed to be closely supervised even when armed with a sharpened pencil.

It certainly seems that in basic training, the practice of medicine is occasionally a trial-and-error exercise, and even the trainees get opportunities to practice. "Some people may have noticed that it tends to get humid in Lackland, Texas, in June," explains Kahlil Ashanti. Humid weather is bad news in any case, but when it is combined with lots of exercise performed in uniforms made of a synthetic material with the permeability of a plastic trash bag, problems will arise—usually with bumps.

"It was inevitable that some people would develop a heat rash, most often on their thighs, which rubbed together whenever they moved. With all the running and marching we did it was like having a fire between your legs. The only cure for it was baby powder, which we all used. So all of us smelled like babies—except for this one person, who didn't understand the basic concept of hygiene. This guy really wasn't very bright, either. So, we sent him to the PX to buy a tube of Vagisil, a product used to treat vaginal funguses. This guy's skin was red, raw, and exposed. When he followed our directions and spread it evenly over the entire inside of his thighs, he waited a few seconds as the area heated—and it was then that he began screaming in pain."

One way to avoid some duty was to ride the sick book, and for some laggards a trip to the infirmary was a day off. Getting there often required more than claiming you don't feel well. You needed an attention-grabber, something that was both unverifiable and odious enough to motivate the medics to get rid of you as soon as possible. As Ira Berkow (army, Ft. Leonard Wood, 1958) recalls, "When we found out that if you went to the infirmary and told them you had diarrhea, they didn't really want to check that you did have diarrhea. This claim did not make our sergeant happy, but there was nothing he could do about it. I told him I had diarrhea, got a sick slip, and was ordered to stay in bed for one day. Naturally I followed orders."

Brian Dennehy went through Parris Island in 1969 with a recruit who also believed diarrhea was his ticket out of the Marine Corps. "In the middle of training he would stop and say, 'Sir . . .' He was driving everybody crazy. Finally the DIs decided they had to deal with him. They had ration boxes, which were like small cardboard shoe boxes. The DI told this kid, 'What you're doing isn't normal. I have been instructed by the medics that you are to collect your shit.' It turned out he meant that literally, continuing, 'I want you to keep these boxes by your bed. Instead of flushing your shit down the toilet, you will collect your shit and put it in a box, then write the time and date on it.' He made another private stay with him when he went to the bathroom to make sure he didn't flush. Not surprisingly, none of this procedure was popular with the rest of the platoon, and the kid gave up and went back to training without any more complaining." This boot made a mistake repeated by many: forgetting that the Drill Instructor was *also* a graduate of basic and in his or her career had encountered just about every attempted trick, deception, artifice, and con at least several times.

Of course, there are trainees for whom basic training is too difficult, who aren't emotionally prepared for the stress, and suicide attempts, while rare, do occur. Trainees have been known to jump off buildings, try to overdose on aspirin, even swallow the Brasso used to shine belt buckles. TI Tim Price had a female "who tried to commit suicide by taking an overdose of Midol. The only thing she succeeded in doing was getting sick to her stomach."

Putting the Fight in the Fighting Man: Hand-to-Hand Combat

HAND-TO-HAND COMBAT INSTRUCTOR AT Ft. Leonard Wood to recruits: "Punch him. Choke him. Kick him in the balls. Gouge his eyes out. Okay! Awwright. Demonstrators relax. And now, the odd numbers will strangle the even numbers."

DRILL INSTRUCTOR: It's freaking hand-to-hand, close fuckin' combat. No freakin' pushing. No freakin' little sister fuckin' love taps. Every blow you throw needs to be like your life freakin' depends on it. Because if you make it, it will . . . You understand that? All the rage and aggression that you have in your body needs to come out on that recruit right there. You don't know him do you? So there's no reason to fuckin' like him is there?

RECRUIT: No Sir!

DRILL INSTRUCTOR: Take out everything you have on that kid right there. You understand? I'm telling you right now, if this were combat, one of you would be going home to your family and one to fucking funeral services. One's going home in a body bag, and one's going home to see his family. Which one are you going to be . . . Why'd you stop? Answer my fucking question before I rip out your teeth. Why'd you stop?

RECRUIT: This recruit thought he heard the whistle, sir.

DRILL INSTRUCTOR: No, you didn't . . . You didn't want to hurt him because you're sweet and nice and you don't want to freaking kill . . . I guess you're going home in a body bag. Don't worry, someone else will take care of your girl.

   —Teaching hand-to-hand combat to Marine recruits from
   the documentary *Ears, Open. Eyeballs, Click.*, directed
   by Canaan Brumley

Homer Hickam remembers, "Hand-to-hand combat was taught in a brutal way. There was nothing fancy about it, it was eye-gouging, stomping, using your combat boots to the best effect, jamming your hand up into your opponent's armpit and busting the arteries in there, using the edge of your hand to attack an opponent's throat; it was just ugly fighting. It wasn't pretty, it wasn't supposed to be, it was just learning how to incapacitate or kill.

"But I do have to say we enjoyed learning how to do it."

Bucks Private: Separating a Recruit and His Pay

As with any large group, at times there are people who are going to take advantage of the situation. As Mitchell Friedman recalls, "The second week of basic training the Bible salesman showed up. Our Drill Sergeants informed us that we were having a competition between units to see which platoon could buy the most Bibles, with the winning platoon getting a weekend pass. The good news was, we were told, that we didn't actually have to pay for them, that the payments could be taken directly out of our pay. At that point a lot of people were really gung-ho, and to show their commitment to the unit they ordered two, even three Bibles." It is hard to see how even guileless recruits could not conclude that they were paying for the Bibles if the money was being taken from their pay, but that is the naivete of young people in the thrall of older ones in leadership positions. In the average assortment of forty youngsters, the law of averages dictates that some will refuse to be lemmings.

"It was so obviously a scam," said Friedman. "There was a group of Jewish recruits from New York, we understood what was going on. They brought us all into the room with the Bible salesman, who had several versions at different prices lined up on a table. We saw right away that there were no Old Testaments there, and we pointed this out to him.

"He said, in a surprisingly friendly tone, 'I ain't got no Kike Bible to show you, and I wouldn't want you to buy one without seeing a sample first.'

"I told him that we had gotten together and agreed that as a group we would buy one Bible for the Day Room! But before we could do that, the Drill Sergeants interrupted and told us that wasn't necessary. As we left, the Bible salesman said in an admiring tone, 'These are the finest Kikes I've ever met.'" Evidently, the Jews weren't the only ones who were alarmed by the enterprise, because several weeks later they marched everyone into the auditorium for an unscheduled session. "The entire cadre was there, every officer, every Drill Sergeant. Whatever this was, it was big. An E-7 stood in front of us and began rambling on about how good the army has been to him, how he owes everything he has to the army, and then finally gets to the point, 'Now if any of you mens did not want to buy a Bible you should have just told us you did not want to buy a Bible, but you really did not have to write to President Nixon.'" For any command, but particularly a training command, a presidential inquiry is among the most labor-intensive, time-consuming, and unpleasant procedures, and the result, as in this case, is often the disciplining of cadre. Making money directly from those over whom you have authority is usually a pretty bad idea, whether God wants you to do it or not.

There are many ways to separate trainees from their property, and it is a sad fact that the honor of serving in uniform does not always translate directly into individual honor. Naive youngsters away from home for the first time, in an alien environment, are often easy marks if they don't recognize quickly that they are the potential prey of people, even superiors, who are less principled.

For example, a popular drill instructor may propose to his recruits that they celebrate his birthday—every single cycle—for which his trainees would collect funds to buy him a present. Or he may ask a trainee if he could "borrow" money until payday, which never seems to come. And unsecured personal items, even toothbrushes, tend to disappear. This is, unfortunately, an age-old story. The night before Joe Salerno reported for training at Ft. Dix in 1943, "My family and friends gave me a money belt and eighty dollars. It was the most money I had ever carried in my life. I got into the barracks at Ft. Dix and we were sleeping in bunk beds. There was an older guy under me, from Newark. 'If you're worried about your money,' he said, 'you know, I'll take care of it for you.' I said, 'No thanks, I'll take care of it.' Well because of what he said I don't think I slept all night. I had my two hands on my belt and I was holding that money."

Although some people are involuntarily separated from their cash and property, others are willing participants in the exercise. For some reason not entirely understood, gambling is particularly popular in the armed forces. It is not unusual that in the barracks after Taps various games of chance tend to appear spontaneously, but troops gamble anywhere and everywhere. During the Second World War, David Jacobs was one of many hundreds of recruits on a train headed west for Camp Crowder, Missouri, to begin basic training, and there was some type of game going on in nearly every car of the train. For David Jacobs, it was dice. The organizer of the game was another recruit who fashioned himself as a big-time gambler, and he must have assumed that Jacobs, who was quiet and spent much of the trip reading, could be an easy mark, but Jacobs refused to play.

The gambler continued to goad him, and finally, to shut the guy up, Jacobs agreed to shoot craps. Having grown up on the streets on Brooklyn, he knew the game, knew it Brooklyn-well, and cleaned him out within fifteen minutes. It was a pretty quiet train ride to Missouri.

Because theft is both common and destructive to morale, instructors will try nearly anything to prevent it and, when it occurs, punish it. Too often it's impossible to identify the thief. While Robert Oxford was at Great Lakes "a guy claimed that $85 was taken from his locker. They told us that no one was going to get liberty, and all of us were going to be kept on our toes and elbows until someone admitted who took the money. No one would admit it so they punished us for hours. That night we went around and collected a dollar from everybody and put it in this kid's locker. Then the kid came out and said his money suddenly reappeared, and so we all got off. That satisfied our instructors, but we never found out who took it."

As in any enterprise, poor or lackadaisical supervision permits any poorly intentioned person to prosper in conducting illegal activities. The patron-sergeant of military scam artists was TV's Master Sergeant Ernie Bilko, the all-time champion of military scam artists. Played by comedian Phil Silvers, Bilko actually drilled for oil in the colonel's basement and was "the only known soldier during the entire conflict of World War II to capture a Japanese prisoner—and hold him for ransom."

In the real world, in places where the leadership is particularly lousy or inappropriate, sometimes criminal behavior can flourish. TI Mike Harrell recalls problems at Lackland in the late 1960s. "We had one guy who was running his own business. He was charging troops for cleaning their sheets or blankets. Some others were charging for liberty. Supposedly, I was working with a Team Chief, although I never saw him. I found out later from my troops that the only time he came around was when he needed money for something, for example to fix his car, and they would take up a collection for him. Basically they were paying him to stay away. I was stunned when I found that out because it meant that I was going to be investigated, too."

Drill Sergeant Michael Johnson had one of his most disheartening experiences literally the night before graduation at Ft. Benning, when one of his trainees discovered that his entire bank account had been emptied. "Early the next morning he went to the bank, and there was a photograph taken by the ATM showing another recruit withdrawing the money. This other guy was someone I had great hopes for. If I had a problem he was the guy I'd want in a foxhole with me. This private had not only taken out the money—he'd made three different attempts. A half hour before graduation I confronted him with the evidence, and he denied it. 'Bullshit, Private,' I told him, 'that's your friggin' face right there.' I almost lost it, but I controlled myself, even though I was so sad and angry. The police came down and arrested him."

What We Have Here Is
a Lack of Communication:
Out of Touch

To prepare people for the potential hardships of military service, to convert them from adolescents into skilled, independent adults, basic training and boot camp instantly and almost completely severs the relationship between trainees and their childhood support groups—family and friends—and builds new adult, professional loyalties.

The advent of new electronic media has made keeping in touch much easier, but it surely isn't the same as hanging around the neighborhood, and for many recruits the worst part of basic training is the loneliness. You're crammed together with dozens of other people, and you're still lonely as hell. No matter how busy you are, you keep thinking about home, and those who are living in a parallel universe without you.

Years ago the only way to communicate with the world outside basic training was by letter or, occasionally, by telephone. Phone calls were prohibited until the later weeks of training—and even then there were only a small number of pay phones anywhere near the barracks, and each of them always had a line of troops waiting impatiently to use it. Pay phone rage often resulted in violent and bloody fights. Occasionally a hapless trainee was designated to keep order, an impossible task. There were few phone lines that didn't eventually produce a broken nose.

As this excerpt from a letter written by twenty-three-year-old Thomas Fenton from New Hope, Pennsylvania, during his first weeks of basic training shows, mail was the only reliable way of keeping in touch with friends and loved ones, making mail call the highlight of every recruit's day—except Sunday:

> March 1942, Biloxi, Mississippi
> Dear Folks and All,
> Got your letter just a few minutes ago and boy was I ever glad. It's the first mail I've got since I left and sure seemed good. Haven't heard from Margie yet, but guess she hasn't had time to get my address and get a letter back. Glad you are all fine and was sorry to hear about the snow. We had a little here but it's about all gone, there's lots of mud and it makes it kinda disagreeable training out on the muddy fields.
> I've written to someone everyday. Didn't write to you yesterday, sure is a lot easier to write after I hear from you. You ask me what I could have. Well, Mom, I can't have much and if you just keep writing so I get lots of mail I'll be satisfied . . .
> Well folks I guess I better kind of sign off and well maybe I better read your letter again maybe I'll write some more. We eat in the morning at 7:00 and at night at 5:30 . . .
> We don't get any mail on Sunday so it's kinda lonesome around here.
> Lots of Love,
> Pvt. Thomas Fenton

Brian Deever said, "My mom had passed away, and it was just me and my father. I didn't expect to get too many letters, because,

I thought, who's gonna to write to me? And the only thing I got from my father was a letter to tell me he wasn't a writer, and so he wouldn't be writing any letters. It was pretty lonely at the beginning, particularly around mail call when I didn't get anything."

Most recruits wrote home whenever they could, sometimes several times daily, and illogically hoped for an immediate response. There are few things that cause dejection more than receiving no mail, especially after you've written dozens of letters. No mail means that for the people back in that parallel universe, you have ceased to exist. Even with the advent of instant communications, the emotional importance of mail call hasn't changed at all for recruits. As Mike Zaleuka wrote late one night, "Lights are out right now, and I'm sitting on the toilet just so I can write this letter. Thank you for all your letters, seriously. I laugh, cry, smile, and frown at them, but they are real, and it's the only real thing I have in my life at the moment. So they are keeping me sane. Dad, you never let me down. Mom, your letters are very calming when I need to take a break . . .

"Tonight was the happiest I have been in . . . forever. I just received six letters. You gave me the fuel to keep going harder and stronger . . . and now I am willing to get up tomorrow morning and work my ass off. Knowing everyone is behind me is very important and I appreciate it."

Perhaps the worst thing any recruit can receive in basic is a "Dear John" letter, in which it is reported that Jody really did get your girl back home. While soldiers have been receiving them since the inception of mail call, they always are painful. Away from home, a trainee's wild imagination sometimes gets the better of him, and in the few idle moments he has to himself, he may imagine all sorts of depressing things, the worst of them being the loss of your love to some Jody. It does happen, and during every cycle several trainees will receive a Dear John letter. Jacob Blizzard (navy, Great Lakes, 2009) explains, "Everyone is so afraid that his girlfriend will forget about them or cheat on them. I was dating someone when I left for boot camp. It was pretty hard because the first two weeks we weren't able to send or receive mail, as if we weren't stressed enough. Some of the guys had never been away from home, and this was really tough on them. By the time we got our first letters it was almost a month. I got a letter from my girlfriend, 'I miss you, I miss you, I can't wait to see you.' I felt great. I was sitting with my rackmate, who slept in the bunk under me, and we were comparing letters. I was raving about how happy I was and I asked him, 'How about you, how's she doing?'

"He had this strange look in his eye and he just said, 'She just broke up with me.' Wow. But some of us were not very sympathetic and made fun of him. The irony was that some of those people making fun of him got their own Dear John letters later in boot camp."

For a long time before the Internet and social media existed, the fastest means of written communication was the telegram. It was an expensive medium, and for a recruit to receive a telegram was a big deal. So often was a telegram used to deliver sad, even devastating, news that Saul Wolfe remembers his own fear when he received a telegram from home. "I had been sent to an area where there was an abundance of dry, hard wax between the crevasses of linoleum tiles, handed a piece of steel wool, and told to clean out those areas. I was on my hands and knees, scrubbing away, when the Drill Sergeant came in. 'Hey Wolfe,' he said. 'You got a telegram. Maybe somebody in your family died.'

"Gees, I thought, and I did get nervous. I opened it up and it read, 'Congratulations! You passed the bar exam. Love Mom and Dad.' That was such great news. I was an attorney! A lifetime of studying had paid off. I drew myself up to full kneeling height, looked up at the sergeant, and said, 'I passed the bar exam!'

" 'That's great,' he said, then indicated the floor. 'Don't miss any spots.' And that was the day I learned humility."

While food and candy are considered contraband, there are times when Drill Sergeants did not intercept them. What could be a greater gesture of love than sending a favorite food from home? Unfortunately, military mail has always has been slow. Milton Pike's parents sent one of Katz's famed salamis to him at Camp Shannon, Texas, in 1944. "And by the time I got it, it was all moldy. I know people think it was the thought that counts, but not when you're away from home, getting ready to go to war. In that situation it was the salami that counted. And this one had to be thrown away."

In any case, even if the food is in good condition—indeed, particularly *because* the food is in good condition—it rarely got eaten by the intended recipient. Dennis Stead, quite overweight and already a prime target of Drill Sergeants, received a two-pound box of chocolates that he *did* get to eat—"immediately. They made me stand there in the center of the room and eat every single piece of chocolate as fast as I possibly could. It was awful, and I made sure no one sent me food again."

Unlike the British, who always treated mail with sanctity—even when broaching it would expose spying and other dangerous activities—in U.S. basic training, nothing is sacred. The public nature of mail call means that there are no secrets. In most units, anyone who received a perfumed letter had to open it and read it out loud, always to the enormous entertainment of the assembled troops. "Boot camp mail call was unique," explains Doug Kasunic (navy, San Diego NTC, 1963). "The entire company of about eighty recruits gathered in a circle surrounding the mail clerk, and he read the addressed names out loud. You couldn't wait to hear your name. The anticipation was tremendous, and so was the disappointment if you didn't get anything. When he called your name, your first thought was: Who was it from? Family? A friend? Your girl? One time I got a letter from a girlfriend who made the mistake of addressing it to 'Douggie Woggie Woo Woo Woo.' Seventynine other people heard the mail clerk call 'Douggie Woggie Woo Woo Woo.'"

Just imagine how unfortunate it is to be among a group of toughened boots when it is revealed that you are known as "Douggie Woggie Woo Woo Woo." Kasunic added, "I can tell you, that was not a good thing to hear yelled out in front of all these tough young guys always looking for a reason to tease someone. And for some reason when it's addressed like that, the mail clerk is going to call it out several times. Loudly. 'Douggie Woggie Woo Woo Woo' was a big hit, and that name stuck with me for four years. How it got from duty station to duty station I'll never know."

Before cell phones existed it was relatively simple for the military to prevent recruits from making phone calls, although some people were known to crawl their way to the phone booth after lights out. On some bases they had a continuing problem replacing the light bulbs in those booths because recruits would smash them to prevent being exposed when they sneaked into the booths, then hunkered down, and shut the doors to make their precious phone calls.

In some army training units, recruits are permitted to call home—once—and to read from a prepared, stilted one-paragraph statement, telling their parents that they had arrived safely at the training base safely and would write soon. That many would not write—sooner or later—is quite beside the point. The military establishment now has responsibility for citizens' children, and the government's most interested customers are the parents of these children. The closing word of the written statement is a simple, "Bye." It has to be read word-for-word, and even small editorial comments—adding 'I love you,' for example—are forbidden and result in push-ups or other punishment.

Cell phones have radically changed the environment. Suddenly a recruit can carry the power of an entire phone booth in a pocket and can furtively call anyone, nearly anytime. Each service has its own policy regarding the use of cell phones, although different army training centers tend to modify the policy in a variety of ways. The Marines do not allow cell phones in boot camp. Period. Conversely, according to official air force policy, trainees "will be authorized to use his/her cell phone to make outgoing calls to family members. Trainees are encouraged to maintain their cell phone service while at BMT. Those arriving without phones will be provided opportunities to utilize pay phones as needed." Trainees at Lackland are told to remove all lewd or pornographic videos. They are limited to a single call each week, lasting a maximum of fifteen minutes and only under the direct supervision of a Training Instructor.

Navy policy has been that phones are to be sent home with the rest of trainees' civilian belongings, but in some units cell phones are kept by instructors and, only on Sundays toward the end of boot camp, the phones are returned to be used briefly.

The army's policy about trainees' use of phones continues to evolve. Robert Hanna reports that in 2005 the policy at Ft. Benning was that phones were forbidden, but by 2010, according to Troy Bayse, "Although during the first half of training at Ft. Benning the only thing we were allowed to do was write and receive letters, once we got out of the first phase, they started letting us get a phone on Sunday for half an hour. Then it became an hour. Later, the policy was that, if we hadn't done anything stupid and we were all working together, the Drill Sergeants gave us back our cell phones and let us use them for a few hours."

Because technology moves more quickly than organizations can change to use it effectively, adaptation is sporadic and uneven. But in 2010 the army began experimenting with actually issuing smart phones to recruits. These devices were loaded with all the information a trainee needs during basic, including a variety of applications including the army manuals, a body fat calculator, and sixteen classic bugle calls. "There were some people who thought this was kind of cheesy," explains former Deputy TRADOC Commander General Mark Hertling, "but this is how young people learn."

Bivouac: A Test of Heavy Mettle

At Fort Knox in the sixth week you go on bivouac, pitching your tent and living like an outdoorsman. You dig foxholes, learn the fundamentals of concealment and camouflage, of scouting and patrolling.

—*Boys Life* magazine, October 1957

THAT BOY'S LIFE DESCRIPTION was not quite the way Joseph Salerno (army, Camp Wheeler, Georgia, 1943) experienced it. "The hardest thing we had to adjust to is the long marches and chiggers. So, me and this kid from New York, we get to the bivouac area, and we're hot. You know, down in Georgia it's hot in July and August. This was our first bivouac, and our sergeant told us, 'Be careful of the chiggers,' but we didn't pay that much attention. Chiggers? We didn't even know what chiggers were. We were hot and sweaty, so we took off our clothes and we laid on the blanket. That turned out to be a mistake. Man, we were so bitten by chiggers that we never did that again. Get into an area, sweat, be uncomfortable, but stay covered!

"The other thing I learned the hard way was when we had to

erect our two-man tents in the field. The sergeant said, 'When you set up your pup tents out in the bivouac area make sure you don't set them up where, if it should rain, the water would accumulate.' My buddy was from New York City and I'm from Newark. So we picked this nice, flat spot at the bottom of a slope. This was a pretty location. Well, it rained that night and formed a creek that ran directly through our tent. We got flooded out. That's how we learned where *not* to put up a pup tent."

At some point during basic training, Marine, army, and even air force recruits spend time living in the field. The navy lives on ships—floating cities, really—and sailors don't have much use for such arcane infantry knowledge as how to dig a slit trench and dispose of human waste, the most successful ways to survive without food, and why it is necessary to march twenty-five miles hauling a sixty-pound pack.

Air force field training became part of Lackland's program in 1942. During the Korean War trainees lived and worked four or five days in an area built to resemble an air base in Korea, not the Ritz by any means, but not an open foxhole at thirty below zero, either. By the 1960s, convinced that no purpose was being served by making trainees miserable just for the purpose of making trainees miserable, the Air Force had completely eliminated bivouacs from training. In 1999, the fifth week of training became known as Warrior Week. This was based on the reality that in the type of wars America is now fighting there is no traditional front line, and every airman may need to know how to survive in the field and fight an armed enemy. In 2008, Warrior Week became (insert ominous music here) known as: the *Beast,* an intense ninety-six-hour combat-zone simulation exercise that requires trainees to put into practice all the skills they had been taught. During the *Beast,* trainees live in a self-contained forward operating base and patrol a 1.5 mile improvised trail that is rife with simulated explosive devices. This is a realistically "deadly" game during which they must find simulated roadside bombs, run and crawl through an obstacle course, and fight an enemy armed with simulated chemical/biological and conventional weapons. The *Beast* is followed a few days later by graduation week, during which each trainee receives his airman's coin and for the first time is addressed as "airman."

Marine boots have to endure "The Crucible," a fifty-four-hour field exercise whose objective is to push trainees to their limits. During the entire duration of the exercises they receive—*in toto*—no more than three meals and eight hours of sleep. They march more than forty-eight miles in full gear and have to fight their way through a series of physical and mental challenges designed to create the greatest amount of stress. Joseph Patrick Bertroche (Marines, San Diego, 2009) explains, "I don't remember much because by the second day I was so dead tired I would black out while marching to a station, and then wake up only because I'd run into the recruit in front of me or stumbled on a rock. Before then, I never thought it was possible to fall asleep while walking.

"We ended up hiking a total of fifty-four miles during the Crucible. We also only got three MREs to eat during the two and a half days. This got especially rough for me at the end because I shared a full MRE with other recruits as they either had theirs stolen or were horrible at conserving food. We got three hours sleep per night; it's supposed to be four but we all had an hour of firewatch."

Training like this is not confined to forcing troops to endure a paucity of food and sleep. If you have ever seen footage of Marines on Iwo Jima, whose fine volcanic sand made advancing under the withering Japanese fire a nearly impossible task, you will have an appreciation for the need to prepare young Marines to this kind of activity. "The first day we got split up into four-man teams," said Betroche, "and had to charge up a heinously steep hill while carrying ammo cans full of sand weighing about thirty-five pounds each. We had to stay aligned with our fire teams all the way up—or we'd have to do it again. Every team ended up doing it at least twice. My team did it three times.

"When we hiked to other stations we'd grab the handle of the recruit's pack in front of us. That sucked because the recruit in front of me was 5'2" so I had to bend way over while power walking three or four miles to the next challenge . . . part of the Crucible was patterned after the Battle of Fallujah. Here it consisted of twelve stations, replicating obstacles in Iraq, such as crossing rivers, evacuating injured Marines, and assaulting through sewers."

The scenario and the teaching points were created by people who had already fought in such circumstances, thus passing along to trainees some of the latest successful techniques learned on the battlefield. Notwithstanding the invaluable experience and professional wisdom of DIs, their freedom of action produced some very odd results, in retrospect both horrifyingly inappropriate and extremely amusing. When David Infante (Marines, San Diego, 1988) went through the Crucible it was "raining cats and dogs with bone-chilling temperatures. We had hiked all day, dug foxholes, and were forced to stay awake for 'fire watch.' Our foxholes filled with water, and the mud was knee deep. In our platoon we had a set of twins who were Native Americans from a reservation. The Drill Instructors called them to their foxholes and ordered them to do a rain dance to make the rain stop. These twins did their thing, but instead of stopping it rained harder. The Drill Instructors got furious and accused the twins of sabotaging the rain dance, doing the one that calls the rain gods to make it rain instead of making it stop."

"There is nothing in the world comparable to the Crucible," according to David Gregory Smith (Marines, Parris Island, 1996). "It's basically three days of survival and land nav. Everything you experience during those three days is designed to create a hardship. You live with whatever you can carry and you have to think about everything you do. Everything counts. I rationed my food minute-by-minute. I would decide, okay, I can have a cracker. I can have a tiny bit of cheese spread now. My entire objective was to save enough food to have my only real meal on the last day." In such circumstances, the honor among comrades is tested as well. Those who were self-centered and morally weak sometimes succumbed to the temptation to steal others' food, but Smith was both disciplined and a pragmatist. "I guarded my food so well," he said, "that on the last day I had enough left to have a full meal. I heated up some beef stew, I made a little place setting for myself and I sat down.

"And there, about sixty filthy, hungry people were staring at me in disbelief. They were practically starving, and I was sitting there with a place setting. It was like being the last live person in *Night of the Living Dead*."

Marvin Dexter (Marines, Parris Island, 2009) was one of those men who did not ration his food. "The Crucible was the most mind-boggling thing I've ever done. I ate all my food on the first day, but I was good, at least until the third day. By the third day there are a lot of hungry, exhausted people. There's some trading for food that goes on; as the day goes on the offers get bigger and bigger!"

A bit like the grueling Boston Marathon, which tests runners with a heartbreakingly torturous hill just when they are the most depleted of energy, the Crucible ends with a long hike. The Reaper, as it is known, consists of climbing four hills and ends with a charge up the final and steepest hill. The top of the rise is not just the finish line of the Reaper and the end of the Crucible, it is also the site of the "Eagle, Globe, and Anchor" ceremony, at which recruits line up and are handed the small, coveted emblem of the Corps. They affix them to their caps, and for the first time in their lives they are addressed as Marines. For the rest of their lives they will be Marines, too.

For its final exam in basic, the army also subjects trainees to a strenuous hike, but the march also integrates the small-unit tactics the trainees learned during the previous eight weeks. Explains Shawn Herbella, "You've done everything else: You've qualified with your rifle, you've passed your PT test, you've done all the exercises and the marches. This is the last thing you have to get through. You pack up all your gear and hike out into the woods. You just walk and walk and walk in two long lines on either side of the road, and along the way, they throw explosions at you, and you have to engage in firefights and other challenges. When you finally get to the end, you dig foxholes, set up a perimeter and go through a variety of tests and drills. After a couple of days of living out there, I was dirty and exhausted—but feeling good."

Surviving the physical demands of basic takes conditioning, but it also requires the ability to control the mind, to get through the difficult moment at hand, and, most of all, to realize that it will not last indefinitely. The Marine Crucible and the army's final FTX are no different in that respect. They are tests designed to be very taxing, but they are also structured so that the large majority of the trainees not only get through them, but actually do very well. There is a great deal of pressure on the individual trainee, but a trainee is best armed against failure when he realizes that there is nothing personal in any of it. Basic is a controlled environment, constantly monitored and then modified at the margins.

Nevertheless, being exposed to the elements offers some perils outside the control of the cadre. Herbella said, "We were staging a mock attack on an enemy position, and it was going well until we ran into a wasp nest. Walking towards an enemy that was shooting at us, as explosions detonated all around us, that was one thing. We were always aware that there was no real danger. Wasps, on the other hand, were different. Wasps stung. Wasps really were dangerous. And these wasps seemed to be especially angry about something. They were stinging us repeatedly right through our clothes. Our Drill Sergeant was telling us, 'Come on, men, we have to force our way through.'

"Right, I thought. Then I turned around and ran the other way." Fighting an enemy trying to kill you is one thing. But wasps? Nobody trains against wasp attacks.

Steven Singer (army, Ft. Polk, 1970) thought his losing battle with insects might be a blessing. "I woke up in the morning and I couldn't close my mouth. My lip had swollen about four times normal size. I could barely speak. Apparently I had been bitten by some type of spider. We were about to begin a seven-mile forced march, and I thought for sure this was my ticket back to Ft. Polk. I went to see the CO. There was drool coming from my mouth, and while it was very hard for me to speak, it was even harder to understand what I was trying to say. I couldn't even tell him that I couldn't talk. The CO couldn't figure out what I was trying to tell him. Finally I got out, 'Ookit my wip.'

"'Oh yeah,' he said. 'You know what? Your lip does look a little swollen. Go to the medical tent and have them give you something to take care of that. But make sure you're packed up first 'cause we're leaving in ten minutes.'

"That's when I figured out the army doesn't march on its lips."

Loaded with every apothecary invention since the dawn of recorded history, military dispensaries have something for everything, and when they don't have what is specifically required, they experiment. With trainees at the peak of their physical lives, there isn't much that goes wrong with them that can't be anticipated. They gave Singer Benadryl, and because the medics sometimes have difficulty with portion control, they gave him way too much. He took what he needed to reduce the swelling, and then traded the rest of it to a recruit as payment for him to shine Singer's boots and make his bunk the last week of basic.

Not all of the exercises on bivouac tested how much trainees had learned, as Tom Mellor (army, Ft. Benning, 1999) found out. "Most of the tasks were job related, but one day they told the whole company to take a shovel and start digging. We dug a hole as big as a swimming pool. When we were done a Drill Sergeant explained, 'Someone took a landmine, a shit in the woods, and didn't bury it, so we're going to have a full military burial for this shit.' They put it in a shoebox and told us to get in the hole with it and show some respect by covering it with dirt. And then while we were all in that hole they threw in some CS gas. I guess it was supposed to be funny. If you were in that hole, it wasn't."

"*Bivouac,*" of course, is a French word, and we use it to mean an encampment, but as with many words in American English, we torture nouns into becoming verbs, and bivouac is no different: A platoon "bivouacs." Originally, the word derived from an Alsatian word, *biwacht* ("by night"), which meant in Napoleonic times a unit that stood guard at night, and that sense is still inherent in establishing a camp. Troops who have been on the march all day, for example, needed to find someplace where they could establish a camp before the sun set, and then set security positions for early warning and defense. Night watch is not effectively established if the unit is stumbling around in the middle of the night. Jo Dawn McEwan (army, Ft. McClellan, 1975) will never forget, "Marching through the swamps at night with artificial bombs going off all around us. It was different than anything any of us had ever experienced. It became real after a while and the next thing I knew we were walking along through those swamps holding hands."

In the field soldiers live in foxholes, which provide protection, allow them to keep ammunition and hand grenades at the ready, and kill the enemy when he attacks. In a defensive combat environment, the most important tools are vigilance and ammo. But when you're not in battle, when you're in an administrative environment, the two most important tools are a shelter half and an entrenching tool.

A shelter half is exactly what it sounds like it is: half of a two-man tent. It comes issued with an assortment of other necessary hardware, including tent poles, tent pegs, and a bit of rope, and when properly erected with your buddy's half, it produces a tiny but perfectly serviceable shelter from the elements. Although the tent is not that difficult to erect, it is annoyingly painful to set it up.

How to set up an army pup tent from two shelter halves:

1. Try to find level ground. Dig a shallow trench around the perimeter to keep rainwater outside the tent. In hot weather try to raise the tent a little higher off the ground to allow more air to circulate.
2. Button two shelter halves together along the top seam only. Spread them on the ground with the front perpendicular to the direction of the wind.
3. Put three tent poles together for the front of the tent. Put the tip of the pole through the metal ring, the grommet, then secure the pole bottom on the ground. Take a guy rope and attach one end to the top of the pole and tie the other end to a stake in the ground. Put a stake through each front tent

stay and pound them into the ground. The stakes should be directed in toward the tent and no more than one inch should be visible above ground. The front of the tent is now assembled.

4. Put three more tent poles together for the back of the tent. Follow the same procedure, stick the pole through the grommet, and pound in stakes to hold it vertical. Now the front and rear of the tent are staked. Stake the sides of the tent.

5. Finally button the front of rear flaps together, but stake down only one side so that one can be opened for cross-ventilation as well as access.

The elaborate procedure is not the only annoyance. The equipment is occasionally balky, incomplete, or frustratingly inappropriate. Saul Wolfe reports that at Ft. Dix in 1958, "Instead of metal tent pegs they gave us wooden pegs. The ground was frozen solid, the pegs would break or split, and so we couldn't hammer them into the ground." However, Wolfe and his buddies discovered, quite by accident, that urinating on the spot softened the ground just enough to sink the pegs. "It was a great discovery," says Wolfe, "except for the part about peeing in that freezing cold weather."

Once a tent has been erected, trainees learn how to camouflage it using natural, local materials. It isn't sufficient merely to tear branches from nearby trees and lay them on the tent. Camouflage is more art than science, and since most people are not particularly artistic, their efforts often result in a tent that looks like somebody tried but failed to camouflage a tent. Some people are very good at it, and for Eric Segal at Ft. Dix in 1966, his camouflage skill presented a bit of a problem. "The whole company put up its tents, and then we camouflaged them. But my partner and I did such a good job that when we returned from chow, we couldn't find our tent. All the tents looked exactly the same to us. We were wandering around and we decided that had to be the best camouflage job ever done."

One of the principal purposes of a tent is to protect its occupants from rain, and shelter halves, like all tents, were made of canvas. This material has an interesting and mysterious but otherwise annoying property. It does a serviceable job of keeping water off the occupants—as long as nothing touches the inside surface of the canvas. A shelter half immediately will begin leaking from any spot you touch. No one seems to know why. It just does. Far too often, trainees learn this through unpleasant experience. They are told repeatedly not to touch the inside of the tent, but it is almost physically impossible for a full-sized soldier with all his equipment to crawl into one of these tents without touching any part of it. Even if he or she does, then the second person has to get in.

There is a related rule: It will rain or snow during bivouac. Invariably. Inevitably. It *always* rains or snows during bivouac. Just as Marty King (army, Ft. Leonard Wood, 1969) and his partner had finished erecting their tent on the top of a hill, a violent thunder and lightning storm erupted. It was a startling experience for two kids from New York City, whose only previous exposure to the elements had been a snowball fight in Central Park. "We didn't know anything about camping, particularly being in the woods during a real storm," said King. "There were trees all around us, and I was afraid one of those trees would get struck by lightning and would fall on our tent. My partner told me he'd read that during a rainstorm snakes will search for the highest and driest ground, which happened to be our tent. So we reached an agreement of shared responsibility: We stayed up all night, and my job was to worry about a tree falling on us, and his job was to worry about snakes crawling into the tent."

Usually, though, it's just the heat or cold, rain or snow. Usually. There are some events that even people experienced in the outdoors can't prepare for. "Our bivouac site was on top of a mountain," Andy McKee (army, Ft. Leonard Wood, 2008) remembers. "We rucked there intending to spend five nights, six days. On the morning of the third day we were sitting around in full gear eating cold waffles as the sun rose. Someone said, 'Look at the sky,' and we all looked up at the same time. The entire bottom half of the sky was a single dark ominous cloud. What was so weird was that the sky above the cloud was an unusual orange. We all said, this can't be good.

"We all stopped eating and just stared at that cloud. One of our Drill Sergeants came out and snapped, 'What the hell are you privates looking at? There ain't nothin' to look at up there.' And then he looked up. 'Oh crap,' he said. 'Everybody get into the tent quick,' he ordered. We all hustled into the tents. They told us to lie on the ground and interlock our arms. We weren't in there two minutes before all hell broke loose. Rain and wind, it was like the world was ending. We were in full gear so all we could do was hold on to our weapons and hope for the best.

"A tornado touched down less than a quarter-mile from our position. There are some things that a pup tent will protect you from, but a tornado isn't one of them. We had no real protection and there was nothing we could have done. We were lucky, that's all, just very lucky."

The End of the Beginning:
The Day the Military Wins

MOST TRAINEES ARE NOT Goldie Hawn's character in *Private Benjamin*. They come to basic training with the understanding that they will be surrendering some—even most—of their liberty. They also hold out some hope that they will be able to maintain at least a small amount of independence, that they would not have to cede complete control of their lives to some overpowering noncommissioned officer. For a time they believe if they play by the rules, follow orders, and don't attract too much attention, they will secretly retain at least the feeling of maintaining control. At some point during basic, they learn just how completely wrong they are. At that point they surrender any concept of self-determination and accept the reality that when they agreed to serve in the armed forces they gave the military absolute control of their lives. They finally accept the fact that unless the orders they are given are immoral or illegal, they will comply with them instantly even if they don't necessarily understand them. They will support them without questioning them. That for their own survival they will do things that they would never have contemplated doing when they were civilians. That's what basic training and boot camp are designed to accomplish, and almost always it succeeds.

That moment at which a trainee finally breaks his bond with civilian life, comes at different times for different trainees, but for quite a few of them, like Ira Berkow (army, Ft. Leonard Wood, 1958), it takes place during bivouac.

"It was about noon. We'd been up since about five o'clock in the morning, and we were starving. We were waiting for the chop drop to deliver food, and it started raining. It was pouring. The truck had to cross a gulley to get to our position, and very quickly that dry gulley became a river. When the food truck tried to cross it, it got stuck. That was our food on that truck! So we got a rope, one guy swam out and tied the rope to the bumper, and we managed to pull the truck up to dry ground."

The troops were so famished that it almost seemed as if they forgot that they were in the midst of a ferocious rainstorm. As if it were a calm and sunny afternoon, they established an orderly chow line, and then proceeded to eat. "They gave us soup and a sliver of beef," says Berkow. "I pulled my poncho over my head and started drinking my soup, but it was raining so hard that the more soup I drank the more I had. I realized I needed to find a dry spot.

"There were no dry spots. We were outside in the rain. I sat against a tree. I had my helmet on my head, covered with my poncho, and my rifle was on my shoulder because they were watching to see if anybody dared put their rifle down. It was unwieldy, and as I reached for my sliver of beef my mess kit tilted and my beef slid off it. I made a grab for it, but I missed. That piece of beef just dropped off the kit and disappeared into the mud. There was nothing else I could do: I plucked the meat out of the mud, cleaned it as best I could, which was basically not at all, and I ate it. That's when I realized they'd won."

Dan Blatt had the same experience at Ft. Dix in 1962. "I don't think I've ever been as cold as I when we were on bivouac. Then it started raining and my clothes got soaked. My roommate had gone on sick call so I was able to lay out my clothes in the tent. When I woke up the next morning all my clothes and my shoes were frozen. For lunch they handed me a hamburger and it fell right on the ground. I didn't even hesitate; I picked it up, brushed off the dirt and ate it. I felt like an animal. That was the moment."

But eventually, bivouac ends. And with it comes an extraordinary sense of satisfaction. "At the end of the bivouac I was filthy, hungry, and exhausted," remembers Shawn Herbella, "and it was one of the proudest moments of my life. There were so many times during those nine weeks that I couldn't believe it was ever going to end. We had a few people run away. They hopped the fence in the middle of the night, and called someone to pick them up, but we'd stuck it out. We'd done it. The feeling was amazing."

The navy doesn't camp out. Its version of a final exam is Battle Stations, an intense twenty-four-hour event that takes place "aboard" the USS *Trayer*, a three-quarter-size "ship in a bottle," a mock-up of a destroyer, located inside a huge building at Great Lakes and sitting in ninety thousand gallons of water. It's so realistic that the wooden pilings on the "pier" to which it's moored even have realistically painted seagull droppings on them. As Casey Gonzales (Great Lakes, 2007) explains, "It's a ship with all types of amazingly realistic Hollywood-style special effects that simulate real battle scenes. In the past recruits would run around the entire base performing tasks, but now it all takes place on this virtual ship. It gets attacked, and you have to respond to all of the situations and problems. It gets hit by a missile, fires break out that you have to fight, holes in the hull have to be plugged, and there are casualties that have to be located and treated. It's like a long, very serious ride at Universal or Disneyworld."

Rooms fill with smoke and water, the boat shakes when it's hit by missiles, sirens scream, the ship loses power, and recruits have to operate in the dark or in red emergency lighting. There are people running all over the place. Battle Stations 21, as it is now known, draws from the lessons learned aboard real ships, ranging from the terrorist attack on the USS *Cole* in Yemen to the disastrous 1967 fire on the aircraft carrier USS *Forrestal*.

It is quite different from the traditional Battle Stations, as conducted before the navy constructed the *Trayer*. That consisted of trainees in full dress, running from station to station to perform very basic tasks. "It was a physically intense confidence course that lasted between twelve and twenty-four hours," reports Philip Landon (Great Lakes, 2005). "We would do things like carrying pipes that we pretended was ammunition from one room to another and making a large pile of those pipes. Then we passed them along, and if we bumped into something or dropped them, we were all theoretically killed in the explosion, and we would have to start building the pile all over again. After that we would go to another room that supposedly was on fire; it was filled with smoke so we couldn't see anything, but our task was to find the wounded dummy in the smoke and carry it out to safety."

Inevitably during exercises whose purpose is to put stress on pretty raw recruits, some of them are going to make mistakes, and it's at the point of difficulty that leadership is most needed and often found. As Jacob Blizzard admits, "After we were supposedly hit by a missile I was assigned to damage control, in charge of a crew that had to patch a hole in the hull. If you can't patch a hole in the side of a ship, you've got a serious problem. Everything around us was so intense that it felt real. Very cold water poured into the room. Okay, I didn't do it exactly right. In fact, I did it completely wrong. If it depended on me, that ship was going down. We were taught that you pack a wooden wedge into the hole with a sledgehammer, more or less creating a cork. But instead of a sledgehammer, I was trying to push the wedge into the hole with my foot. I was kicking it as hard as I could. It wasn't happening.

"Fortunately, one of my shipmates pushed me aside and said, 'I got this one, I got this.' He used the sledgehammer and saved that ship for us."

"I screwed up," Chris Sergeant (Great Lakes, 2010) also admits. "During Battle Stations they don't tell you how to solve a problem, but sometimes, if you're really not getting it, they do give you hints that you're doing something wrong. We were moving munitions from one magazine to another. As a magazine loaded with munitions was filling with smoke and we were all standing around worrying what to do about it, one of the hints was, 'Standing around in a room filled with ammunition about to burst into flame doesn't seem like a real good idea. You might want to get out of this room and start moving the munitions somewhere else.'"

"I messed up," Will Cortez (Great Lakes, 2010) says. "To be honest I just panicked. There is a part of damage control in which you have to rescue a wounded person from a room that's on fire, filled with smoke. They use 130-pound dummies that actually moan and cry. This was the first time we'd been without our division trainers. Battle Stations starts slow, standing watches, taking the ship out, normal stuff, but at the end it gets really intense really fast. That room was on fire and filling with smoke. I couldn't see anything. We were running out of time looking for that casualty. Finally I said, 'I can't find him, let's get out of here. We're wasting time.' That was a bad decision on my part, but it was an important lesson that I learned."

The day they arrive at boot camp navy trainees are handed a baseball cap that reads "recruit" which they wear throughout the cycle, but to mark the successful conclusion of Battle Stations they're handed a ball cap reading "Navy," and for the first time are addressed as sailors.

Graduation follows a few days later, as Scott Hunt (Great Lakes, 2009) describes it, "We marched into the Great Hall, which is like a giant auditorium with bleachers. As you march in those bleachers are filled with family and friends and the feeling is indescribable. I felt like I was the lead singer of Led Zeppelin playing a concert in downtown London in front of half the population of England. Your heart opens up, you got goose bumps, and you feel that this is what life is all about."

No one graduates from basic training or boot camp the same person they were when they arrived. "Most of the people I came with to basic training were college graduates," remembers Saul Wolfe. "We were going to retain our independence. During the Korean War the army had had a lot of problems so they were teaching us the Code of the American Fighting Man, and part of it is, 'I will never surrender.'

"Being college educated, some of us had even attended law school, we felt the need to be accurate, so we said, 'I will never surrender so long as I have the means to resist.'

"The Drill Sergeants were adamant, 'No, it's I will never surrender.'

"But we had the college degrees and they didn't, so we insisted it was correct to say 'I will never surrender as long as I have the means to resist.'

"And they were the Drill Sergeants who had the power. 'Okay, give me fifty push-ups, now run around the building a few times, and let's try to say it correctly.'

"At first we really did believe we would get through it without really becoming a soldier. We were reservists, we knew it was only temporary. It took us awhile to figure it out. Our Drill Sergeant would take us into a muddy field and order, 'When I tell you to hit it, you don't hesitate. You hit it.' When he screamed 'Hit it,' we would look around for a dry spot or a soft spot so we wouldn't get too dirty or it wouldn't hurt too much, and eventually we'd get down. Too slow. So he ordered us to do it again, and again, faster, over and over, we hit it and hit it and hit it until we just were too tired to resist. Then we hit it some more, did some push-ups, ran around, marched with full packs and when he said hit it, we hit it right into the mud. We became exactly what they wanted us to become. While we were on parade in our dress uniforms at the graduation ceremony marking the end of basic training I was convinced that if someone had yelled 'Hit it' every single one of us would immediately be on the ground burying our face in the dirt."

After being drafted Gene DeSantis (army, Ft. Jackson, 1966) tried everything to get out of basic. "I went to sick call all the time to complain about my bad back. I even wrote to my congressman and the army's chief surgeon examined me and said I was fit for duty. Then after several weeks I got with the program. By the time I finished my training I was so freaking gung-ho that I felt on top of the world. I ended up fulfilling my obligation, getting a commission, and signing up for another two years."

Mike LaRoche finished basic training at Ft. Benning in 2004 "believing I could take on anything they threw at me. I had learned a lot about myself, what I could handle and where I needed help. I don't know how much more mature I became, but I did gain some sense of maturity. But the biggest thing for me was that my level of self-confidence was through the roof!"

When Steve Baudo went into the air force in 1964 admittedly he "had no focus in life. I graduated high school and didn't have the slightest idea what to do next. It was in basic training that I became a man. I learned to be responsible for my actions, to value my integrity, to take care of myself, and how to fold my clothes and roll my socks. It gave me the foundation that I needed for the rest of my life."

"When I left for basic training," Peter Flood (army, Ft. Dix, 1968) remembers, "I told my friends, 'If I ever say I got anything good out of this, just shoot me.' I think I was too young to understand that I was in trouble in my life. I had a lot of freedom but I didn't exercise a lot of responsibility. Within a couple of weeks I was writing letters to people saying I was completely wrong. In basic I was introduced to a world in which you either functioned or failed. The ability to succeed was left completely up to you, this was an opportunity to be as good as you were willing to be. At that time my life had no structure and I was self-limited. Being transported to a place where structure was imposed by people who knew exactly what they were doing turned my life around. Absolutely."

Marine Corps boot camp gave Brian Dennehy "the confidence that has done me a lot of good over the years. I learned how much I could take, which was a hell of a lot more than I originally believed." Ira Berkow learned in army basic training "that I could do things I hadn't imagined I could do. I would say it was nine weeks of hell but as the years passed and I ran into obstacles I would think to myself, you got through basic training, you sure as hell can get through this."

One more thing often happens at the end of basic training: The cadre turns out to be human. "The day after we graduated," Tom Seaver (Marines, San Diego, 1962) recalls, "our Drill Instructor got everyone together. He'd been very rough on us, but the day we became Marines that all changed. He was sitting around talking to us. We knew he'd been awarded a Silver Star, but he'd never spoken about it. One of the new Marines finally asked him how he'd earned it, and he said quietly, 'If you wanted to know, you should have been there.'

"Ten years later I happened to run into him. By this time I was pitching in the major leagues, but the instant I saw him I was transported back to boot camp. I recognized him immediately and told him that I had been in a platoon he'd trained. 'Are you serious?' he asked.

"'Absolutely,' I said, reeling off my serial number. 'It changed my life.' And when he asked me how I recognized him so quickly I had to laugh, 'You got stuck in my brain.'"

As Congressional Medal of Honor recipient Sammy Lee Davis says, "I thought my Drill Sergeant, Sergeant Francisco Corones, hated me. He picked on me relentlessly, and he was always in my face. But the night before we graduated he called me into his room and said, 'Sit down, Sam.'

"I wondered what this was all about. I thought I was finally done with him. Then he pulled out a bottle of Old Crow, handed me the bottle, and told me, 'Have a sip. Look, I know I've been harder on you than some of the other men, but there was a reason for it. I know you had more potential and I wanted to bring it out of you.' And he did. He certainly did."

When Mike Volkin left Ft. Leonard Wood after finishing basic training in 2001 he also believed he'd left behind a Drill Sergeant he had grown to hate. "This was a terrible individual. He was on my back the whole time, and by the time we were done I couldn't stand him. I was at the airport in St. Louis waiting for my plane home when I heard this voice shouting, 'Specialist Volkin.' I recognized his voice immediately and my whole body tensed up. I thought I was done with him.

"I turned around and he was at the other end of the hallway, and he shouted loudly enough for everybody to hear, 'You did a good job, Specialist. You did it very well. Nice going.'

"I said, 'Thank you,' and then I turned away from him. Maybe he wasn't such a bad guy."

INDEX

INDEX

INDEX

INDEX

INDEX